AF718661

Medicine & Society In America

Medicine & Society In America

Advisory Editor

Charles E. Rosenberg
Professor of History
University of Pennsylvania

Psychanalysis

Its Theories and Practical Application

BY

A. A. BRILL, Ph.B., M.D.

ARNO PRESS & THE NEW YORK TIMES

New York 1972

Reprint Edition 1972 by Arno Press Inc.

Copyright © 1912 by W.B.Saunders Company
Reprinted by permission of
Gioia B. Bernheim and Edmund R. Brill

LC# 78-180559
ISBN 0-405-03939-5

Medicine and Society in America
ISBN for complete set: 0-405-03930-1
See last pages of this volume for titles.

Manufactured in the United States of America

Psychanalysis

Its Theories and Practical Application

BY

A. A. BRILL, Ph.B., M.D.

Chief of the Neurological Department of the Bronx Hospital and Dispensary; Clinical Assistant in Psychiatry and Neurology at Columbia University Medical School; formerly Assistant Physician to Central Islip State Hospital, and to the Clinic of Psychiatry, Zurich

PHILADELPHIA AND LONDON

W. B. SAUNDERS COMPANY

1913

Copyright, 1912, by W. B. Saunders Company

Reprinted May, 1913

PRINTED IN AMERICA

PRESS OF
W. B. SAUNDERS COMPANY
PHILADELPHIA

TO MY ESTEEMED TEACHER

PROFESSOR DR. SIGMUND FREUD, LL. D.

WHOSE IDEAS ARE HEREIN REPRODUCED THIS

BOOK IS AFFECTIONATELY INSCRIBED

PREFACE

Like many others in the field of nervous and mental work, I received my training in the State Hospital for the insane. It was my fortune to enter the hospital service at a very important period of its development. Dr. Frederick Peterson was then president of the Commission in Lunacy, and it was mainly through his untiring energy that the New York State hospitals were thoroughly modernized and put on a firm scientific basis. It was also mostly through his efforts that Dr. Adolf Meyer became director of the Pathological Institute at Ward's Island, N. Y.

The advent of Dr. Meyer marks a new epoch in the N. Y. State hospital service. An accomplished neuropathologist and psychiatrist of long experience, he soon instilled new life and interest into the work by giving regular courses of lectures and demonstrations to the internes on the theories and methods then in vogue. The old way of writing a one line note about the patient's mental and physical condition every three or six months had to stop despite the grumbling of the "old timers," and we were required to make frequent and comprehensive examinations of our patients and note carefully what we found. These examinations were made in accordance with a scheme thoroughly worked out by Dr. Adolf Meyer, the underlying principles of which were the teachings of Kraepelin, Wernicke and Ziehen. This good work has continued up to the present with excellent results. Since

I left the state service I have visited and worked in some of the best psychiatric clinics in Europe, and I am glad to say that all things considered the work of the New York State Hospital compares very favorably with the work done in most of the hospitals of its kind.

What I say in reference to the N. Y. State hospitals can be readily applied with some modifications to most of the hospitals for the insane in this country. It is well known that within the last ten to twelve years the management and treatment of the insane in this country have undergone a marked transformation, which is of great benefit to the patient, the doctor and the public. The State hospitals are now treating the patients as patients in the true sense of the word; they are rapidly filling up an enormous gap in the medical profession by training doctors how to treat the insane, and they are gradually abolishing the popular prejudices against hospitals for the insane. The medical schools, too, are now paying more though not enough attention to mental diseases; and last, but not least, excellent and commendable work is being done by the Social Service Departments and the National Society for Mental Hygiene.

The progressive evolution in the study of mental diseases has called attention to another neglected field in which the most important work is still to be done. I refer to the so-called "borderline" cases, the neuroses and mild psychoses who never reach the State hospitals, but form the greatest proportion of clinic and dispensary practice. In the ten years from 1900–1909, 21,290 patients were examined by the assistants in the neurological department of the Vanderbilt Clinic, N. Y., and about 25% of this number were diagnosed as neurasthenia, psychasthenia, hysteria, and as mild forms of the functional psychoses.[1] Although I am not ready to give statistics, I do not hesitate to assert that the same conditions prevail in almost every clinic and dispensary. A striking feature in these borderline cases is the fact that the great majority run a chronic course. Up to within recent years no real effort has been made to understand these unfortunates. It is gratifying to note, however, that a complete change has taken place in this direction. Physicians now realize that the old adage *mens sana in corpore sano* is not to be taken in the strict sense, and hence do not rely on physical treatment alone. All enlightened and progressive physicians recognize psychotherapy as an important therapeutic agent in the treatment of these borderline cases of mental diseases.

Now as there is a demand for psychotherapy, the question naturally arises as to which is the method of preference. Without entering into the merits and demerits of the different systems of psychotherapy, admitting that in competent hands they are all good and useful, and that I myself employ them in certain cases, I do not hesitate to assert that psychanalysis is the most rational and effective method of psychic therapy. I say this after I have practised for years the existing psychotherapeutic methods. Psychanalysis is the only system of psychotherapy that deals with the neuroses as entities instead of treating symptoms, as do hypnotism, suggestion and persuasion. To hypnotize a patient because he suffers from obsessions or phobias is equivalent to treating the cough or fever

[1] Jelliffe and Brill: Statistical Summary of Cases in Department of Neurology, Vanderbilt Clinic, for Ten Years, 1900 to 1909, Journal Nervous and Mental Diseases, July, 1911.

regardless of the disease of which it is but one of the manifestations. Hypnotism takes no cognizance of personality, it simply imposes blind obedience which at best lasts until worn off. Psychanalysis always concerns itself with the individual as a personality and enters into the deepest recesses of the mind. It is for that reason that the results of psychanalysis are most effective; and it is only through psychanalysis that we can hope to gain a real insight into the neuroses and psychoses, a thing of prime importance in the study of mental prophylaxis.

These assertions are not based merely on the reading of a few scattered papers, but on about six years of hard work and almost constant occupation with the subject. For it is only through hard work and long experience that one can acquire a thorough knowledge of Freud's psychology. Recently I had the pleasure of talking to some who claimed to have used psychanalysis in the treatment of patients, and who spoke rather discouragingly, saying that it produced no result. Thus one endeavored to cure a case of so-called congenital homosexuality in about a dozen sessions. Another stated that although he questioned a young woman for hours about sex she showed no improvement in her hysteria.

Such statements readily show the gross misunderstanding of the work. For it is not the treatment of a few hours, weeks or even months that cures; it is the psychic elaboration accomplished during a long period by one thoroughly conversant with the work. I do not think that it is too much to ask of one who wishes to make use of a certain technical method that he should first learn its basic principles. One cannot expect to become proficient in psychanalysis unless he has mastered at least

Freud's theories of the neuroses, the interpretation of dreams, the sexual theories, the psychopathology of everyday life, and his book on wit, and last but not least who has not had a training in nervous and mental work. Besides these qualifications one must know how to select his cases. It has been wrongly supposed that we claim to be able to cure everything. Neither Freud nor any of his pupils has ever advanced such claims. On the contrary, Freud has repeatedly emphasized that psychanalysis has a limited field, and that it should be used only in limited cases. Let us hear what he says:

"The former value of the person should not be overlooked in the disease, and you should refuse a patient who does not possess a certain degree of education, and whose character is not in a measure reliable. We must not forget that there are also healthy persons who are good for nothing, and that if they only show a mere touch of the neurosis, one is only too much inclined to blame the disease for incapacitating such inferior persons. I maintain that the neurosis does not in any way stamp its bearer as a dégenéré, but that, frequently enough, it is found in the same individual associated with the manifestations of degeneration. The analytic psychotherapy is, therefore, no procedure for the treatment of neuropathic degeneration, on the contrary it is limited by it. It is also not to be applied in persons who are not prompted by their own suffering to seek treatment, but subject themselves to it by order of their relatives.

"If one wishes to take a safe course he should limit his selection to persons of a normal state. Psychoses, confusional states, and marked (I might say toxic) depressions, are unsuitable for analysis, at least as it is practised to-day. I do not think it at all impossible that with the proper changes in the procedure it will be possible to disregard this contraindication, and thus claim a psychotherapy for the psychoses.

"The age of the patient also plays a part in the selection for the psychoanalytic treatment. Persons near or over the age of fifty lack, on the one hand, the plasticity of the psychic processes upon which the therapy depends—old people are no longer educable—and on the other hand, the material which has to be elaborated and the duration of the treatment are immensely increased. The earliest age limit is to be individually determined; youthful persons, even before puberty, are excellent subjects for analysis.

"One should not attempt psychoanalysis when it is a question of rapidly removing a threatening manifestation, as, for example, in the case of an hysterical anorexia."[1]

From my own experience I fully agree with Freud, and I would add: do not analyze your relatives, and when in private practice do not analyze any patient without receiving some compensation for it.

As the actual working method will be described later, I shall confine myself here to a few facts, which, although strictly speaking belong to the epilogue, may nevertheless be worth mentioning in this connection. With the beginning of the analysis I investigate the patient's dream life. I instruct him to write down his dreams on awakening. This is very important because dreams give us the most reliable information concerning the individual, and they

[1] Freud: Selected Papers on Hysteria and other Psychoneuroses, 2d Ed., p. 181. Trans. by A. A. Brill, Jour. Ner. and Men. Dis. Pub. Co.

invariably show some relation to the symptoms. I never attempt, however, to analyze a dream before knowing the patient for at least two weeks. Dreams cannot be analyzed unless one has the full cooperation of the dreamer, and this is only possible after a certain *rapport* has been established between the doctor and the patient.

It is this *rapport*, or the transference[1] as we will call it, with which one must start. Nothing can be done without it, and unless this is properly managed little can be done for the patient. One may get excellent results in surgery or in any other specialty without seeing the patient's face, but psychanalysis presupposes an intimate acquaintanceship. There must be a mutual understanding and liking between doctor and patient. One must, however, be on his guard lest the transference be carried too far. One must remember that one is dealing with people whose libido strives for fixation, and care and tact must therefore be exercised to remain good friends only. One must remember the intimate relationship existing between love and hatred, and that one can be readily changed into the other. There are few neurotics, or for that matter normal beings, who remain absolutely indifferent. They either like or dislike. In one of his essays, Charles Lamb tells of two men who never met before who began to fight as soon as they saw each other. This sounds very strange to us, though it is comprehensible in savages, children and animals. As is known, neurotics are dominated by

[1] Freud: Zur Dynamik der Übertragung, Zentralb. f. Psychoanalyse, 2. Jahrgang, Heft 1 und 4. Stekel: Die verschiedenen Formen der Übertragung, Zentralb. f. Psychoanalyse, 2. Jahrgang. Ferenczi: Introjection und Übertragung, Jahrbuch f. Psychoanalyt. u. Psychopath., 1910, Bd. i, p. 451. Jones: The Action of Suggestion in Psychotherapy, Jour. of Abnormal Psychol., January, 1910.

their infantile or repressed material, they suffer from a failure in repression; hence behave in a way like children.

It is hardly necessary to mention that we are criticised for delving into sexuality. This is quite true, but it is a question whether it merits criticism. Our critics seem to have no conception of Freud's idea of sexuality. To us the term is very broad, it really comprises the whole love-life of the individual. As soon as we enter into the intimate life of the patient we are sure to find sex in some form, and the best indication of an abnormal sexual life is an apparent absence of the sexual factors. It is naturally advisable to be very careful in approaching the subject so as not to shock the patient. Moreover, psychanalysis presupposes a knowledge of not only Freud's theories of sex, but also a broad knowledge of psychosexuality in general. Only those who are themselves free from all sexual resistances and who can discuss sex in a pure-minded manner should do psychanalytic work.

In conclusion I wish to say that the main object of this book is to present the practical application of Freud's theories in one volume, hoping thereby not only to remove many false conceptions entertained concerning psychanalysis, but to stimulate further interest in Freud's original works.

As some of the material given here has been published before in the Journal of Abnormal Psychology, the American Journal of Insanity, the N. Y. Medical Journal, the Medical Record, and the N. Y. State Journal of Medicine, I take this opportunity to express my thanks to the editors of these journals for allowing me to utilize the same.

A. A. BRILL.

NEW YORK CITY.

CONTENTS

PSYCHANALYSIS

ITS THEORIES AND PRACTICAL APPLICATION

CHAPTER I

THE PSYCHONEUROSES

The Development of Freud's Conception of the Psychoneuroses and Psychoses, Their Relation to the Psychology of Dreams, Sex and the Psychopathology of Every-day Life

The psychoneuroses, the step-children of medicine, have of late received more attention in the literature than before. Both here and abroad it has been realized that there is a large group of diseases, the so-called border-line cases in mental diseases, the understanding and treatment of which has been sadly neglected, and it is gratifying to know that at least some steps have been taken to meet these deficiencies. The wave of psychotherapy which has swept the continent has also made its presence felt in this country through its numerous discussions in both lay and professional journals. Abroad its adherents claim brilliant results; one need only review the numerous works of the Nancy and other schools to be convinced that psychotherapy is no empty term, but an actual branch of medicine, and that in the psychoneuroses it is the only effective remedial agent.

Yet, whereas all schools agree that the psychoneuroses should be treated by psychotherapy, they all disagree as to the nature of the psychoneuroses. One need only scan the recent works to see that diverse views are expressed by the different investigators on the subject. These diversities, in my opinion, are due to the fact that most of the investigators in question have ignored one important factor, namely, individual psychology. Without individual psychology the riddle of the neuroses, like the riddle of the psychoses, must remain unsolved.

Among the different views expressed on the neuroses those of Freud stand out most conspicuously. No recent theories in medicine or psychology have evoked so many controversies and discussions. After years of careful and painstaking labor Freud evolved not only a system of psychotherapy, but a new psychology. Unlike all other investigators he discarded all generalities and confined himself to the individual. The individual factors which had escaped the notice of other investigators he found to be of the utmost importance in the psychogenetic development of personality.

As early as 1895 Breuer and Freud published the "Studien über Hysterie." They found that hysterical symptoms like neuralgias, paralyses, epileptiform attacks, etc., could be traced to actual psychic traumata which the patient could not consciously recall, but which could be readily demonstrated when the patient was put in the hypnotic state. In other words, they found that the hysterical manifestations were not accidental, but had an actual cause. The connection between cause and effect was often quite obvious; thus, "A very sick child falls asleep and the mother exerts all her will power to make no noise to awaken it, but just because she resolved to do so she emits a clicking sound with her tongue (hysterical counter-will) which was repeated on another occasion when she wished to be absolutely quiet. This developed into a regular tic which lasted for years."[1] In some cases the connection is not so simple, there being only a symbolic relation between the cause and the hysterical phenomena; thus, psychic pain may cause a neuralgia and moral disgust may cause vomiting. Breuer and Freud then concluded that these psychic traumata, or the memory of the same, act like foreign bodies in consciousness, and even long after their occurrence continue to influence like causative factors; to quote Freud, "The hysteric suffers mostly from reminiscences."[2] Their symptoms are remnants and memory symbols for certain (traumatic) events. A deeper understanding of these symbolisms will perhaps be gained by comparing them with memory symbols of other spheres. Thus the statues and monuments with which we embellish our big cities are such memory symbols. "If you should take a walk through London you would find a richly decorated Gothic column in front of Charing Cross, one of the largest railroad stations of the city. On the occasion of removing to Westminster the remains of his beloved queen, Eleanor, one of the old Plantagenet kings in the XIII century ordered that Gothic crosses be erected at every station where the funeral procession halted, and Charing Cross is the last of the monuments commemorating this funeral procession. In another place in the city not far from London Bridge you will notice a modern lofty column which is briefly referred to as 'The Monument.' It is supposed to commemorate the big fire which started near there in 1666 and destroyed a large part of the city. These monuments, therefore, like the hysterical symptoms, are memory symbols. So far the comparison is justified. But what would you think of a Londoner who would even to-day halt in grief before the monument of the funeral procession of Queen Eleanor instead of continuing on his way with the required haste of modern business conditions? Or what would you think of another who would stop before 'The Monument' and bewail the conflagration of his beloved native city? Yet hysteric and neurotic individuals behave exactly like these two impractical Londoners. Not only do they recall the long forgotten painful events, but they stick to them with all their emotions. They cannot get away from the past and neglect for it reality and the present. This fixation of the psychic life on the pathogenic traumas is one of the most important, and, from a practical viewpoint, one of the most significant characters of the neurosis."[3]

That the hysterical symptoms are only reminiscences was proven by the fact that the individual hysterical symptoms disappeared without returning if one succeeded in thoroughly awakening the memories of the causal process with its accompanying affects and if the patient circumstantially discussed the process, giving free play to the affect. The reason for the strangulation of the emotion was because at the time of its occurrence it could not be adequately worked off. We all know that it is not always possible to give vent to our feelings, and that an insult retaliated leaves quite a different impression than one that has to be swallowed.

The treatment called "catharsis" consisted in reconducting the sum of excitement from its false paths to the original conscious idea and then working it off by means of intellectual labor and speech. The patient was hypnotized and questioned about the origin of the symptoms and while recalling the original injuries, either in hypnosis or the normal state, the hemmed-in emotions were discharged and the symptoms disappeared. This is the so-called "abreagirung"—abreaction—which means to work off something by living through it again. It was noticed that the affect appeared with special intensity during the reproduction of the scenes which gave origin to the symptom and completely disappeared with their termination. On the other hand, no result was noticed when the scenes evoked were not accompanied by any emotional feeling.

This is rather a brief review of the conceptions originally expressed by Breuer and Freud. It is from these principles that Freud developed his present conceptions of the psychoneuroses and his revolutionary psychology.

When Freud continued to practice his cathartic treatment he was confronted with one special difficulty. He found that not all persons were hypnotizable and as hypnosis was absolutely essential for the broadening of the patient's consciousness, many patients had to be given up as they could not be hypnotized. He even went so far as to take one of these patients to Nancy to Bernheim, but after applying all his skill Bernheim had to admit that he, too, could not hypnotize the patient.* This and a number of other reasons caused Freud to avoid hypnotism and to adopt a new procedure which he calls the psychoanalytic method. On asking the patients in the waking state whether they remembered the first motive of the symptom in question, some knew nothing while others recalled something rather vaguely. Freud then applied the same method which Bernheim used in awakening the manifestly forgotten impressions produced during somnambulism. He found that by urging and assuring the patients that they did remember and telling them that all they had to do was to concentrate their attention, and repeat the thoughts which would occur to them they finally recalled the pathogenic ideas without hypnotism. But as this urging necessitated much exertion on his part, and showed him that he had to overcome great resistance in the patient, he formulated the following theory: "Through my psychic work I had to overcome a psychic force in the patient which opposed the pathogenic idea from becoming conscious."[4] The resistance was due to the fact that the ideas which had to be disinterred were all of a nature adapted to provoke the affects of shame, reproach, mental pain and a feeling of injury—they were altogether of that kind which one would not like to experience, and prefers to forget.

This gave rise to Freud's idea of repression; the pathogenic idea being of a painful nature is incompatible with the ego, and is therefore treated by it as *non-arrivé*. The patient wishes to know nothing about it, he wishes

* That not every person can be hypnotized has been long acknowledged by all experienced observers of the subject.

to forget it. But as this repression, or forgetting, never succeeds completely, the pathogenic idea continues to strive to come to the surface, and is constantly inhibited by the psychic censor. This struggle of the two opposing forces results in a compromise. Each foregoes a part of the original demand, thus meeting the other half way, and the result of this mutual accommodation is then transformed into a hysterical symptom by the process of *conversion*. In this manner the ego frees itself from opposition, the original painful idea or unattainable wish is forgotten, and instead it becomes burdened with a memory symbol which remains in consciousness as an unadjusted motor or sensory innervation. We thus see that the main character of hysteria is not the splitting of consciousness as asserted by Janet and his school, but the ability of converting the sum of strangulated emotion either totally or partially, into that motor or sensory innervation which is more or less connected with the traumatic event. In brief the study of the psychoneuroses shows conclusively that there was a failure in the repression of the idea concerning the unattainable wish. To be sure the painful idea is crowded out of consciousness and memory and the individual thus spares himself a great deal of pain, but the repressed wish remains in the unconscious and lurks for an opportunity to become active. When it succeeds it brings to the surface a distorted and strange substitutive formation which soon becomes connected with the same pain the individual got rid of through the repression. This substitutive formation is the symptom and in hysteria it is produced by the process of conversion.

There are, however, predisposed persons in whom there

is no adaptation for conversion. Here, if an unbearable idea enters consciousness it meets with the same contrary forces as those mentioned above, the affect becomes detached from the idea, but instead of being converted into the physical, it remains in the psychic sphere. The weakened unbearable idea remains apart from all association in consciousness, but its detached affect or the sum of excitement allies itself to another indifferent idea,[5] which on account of this "false" connection becomes an obsession; or the unbearable idea is so changed that the patient does not recognize it. He no longer thinks of the painful or disagreeable, but instead he is burdened with an obsession, the absurdity of which he realizes, but from which he cannot rid himself. The advantage thus gained by the ego in the transposition or dislocation of the affect is not as great as in the hysterical conversion of psychic excitement into somatic innervation. The affect remains unchanged and undiminished, but the unbearable idea is suppressed from memory.

The same mechanism holds true for the origin of phobias, and both come under the heading of compulsion neurosis. It was also found that the unbearable ideas underlying the compulsion neurosis (obsessions, doubts and phobias) have their origin in the sexual life. In the words of Freud, "the obsession represents a compensation or substitute for the unbearable sexual idea and takes its place in consciousness."[6]

Both hysteria and compulsion neurosis belong to the defense neuropsychoses; their symptoms originate through the psychic mechanism of defense, that is through the attempt to repress a painful idea which was incompatible with the ego of the patient. In both neuroses the idea is robbed of its affect, and excluded from associative elaboration, remaining, however, in consciousness.

There is still another far more forceful and more successful form of defense, wherein the ego misplaces the incompatible idea with its emotion and acts as though the painful idea had never come to pass. When this occurs the person merges into a psychosis which may be called "hallucinatory confusion." To illustrate this form of defense I will cite a case which, through the kindness of Dr. M. S. Gregory, I saw in the psychopathic pavilion of Bellevue Hospital. It concerned a young married man of about thirty years, a New Yorker, who, being out of work, tried his fortune as a farm-hand up the state. Things did not go as smoothly as he expected, and one day the farmer gave him a rather severe thrashing, and dismissed him without paying him his salary. He sought redress, but could get none so that he had to walk to New York City penniless. When he returned home he made a number of attempts to obtain justice for himself, but was told that he could do nothing. He kept on brooding over it for some time, when one day he suddenly became excited and confused. He became boisterous, cursing the farmer, and accompanied his utterances by violently kicking the bedstead and the pillows. He imagined that he was punching the farmer. He was so excited and confused that his wife sent for the police who took him to the psychopathic pavilion of Bellevue Hospital.

Here the idea was so painful that the ego tore itself away from it, but as the painful idea was inseparably connected with reality the ego had to exclude itself wholly from reality. Such cases give us an insight into the psychoses. Thanks to the genius of Freud and the Zurich school[7] we no longer fear to face the hitherto considered perplexities of the insane mind. As will be shown later every insane utterance, every morbid perception, has a definite meaning and a definite *raison d'être* when analyzed. Truly there is method in madness.

In tracing the psychic traumas which are supposed to be at the basis of hysterical symptoms or compulsion neuroses, one invariably comes to sexual experiences of childhood. This is so conspicuous that it led Freud to lay great stress on the sexual and to formulate the following sentence: "In a normal vita sexualis no neurosis is possible."[8] This, I know, sounds rather strange, but I would like to call attention to the fact that the sexual impulse is one of our strongest impulses. It is the one impulse that is subjected to the greatest amount of repression and for that reason it has always been the weakest point in our cultural development. It must also be borne in mind that Freud's conception of the sexual is very broad. It is just as broad as our English word "love" or the Greek word "eros," and does not at all limit itself to the gross sexual. Moreover, it must be remembered that sexuality is more complicated than one thinks. Hypocrisy and prudishness have from time immemorial tabooed all things sexual; the word itself carries with it the ideas of lewdness and loathing. As a result of this the ignorance displayed in matters sexual is appalling. Thus we are led to believe that there is no sexuality before a certain age, the age of puberty, yet when we look back to our own youth we find that long before that age we were subjected to certain feelings which were unmistakably of a sexual nature. Freud maintains that the sexual is born with us and begins to manifest itself in infancy. "It seems certain," he says, "that the newborn child brings with it the germs of sexual feelings which continue to develop for some time and then succumb to a progressive suppression, which is, in turn, broken through by the proper advance of sexual development and which can be checked by individual idiosyncrasies."[9] He also tells us that the sexual impulse in man consists of many components and partial impulses. Many essential contributions to the sexual excitement are furnished by the peripheral excitement of certain parts of the body, such as the genitals, mouth, anus and bladder outlets. All these zones are active in infancy and only some of them go to make up the sexual life. The first libidinous manifestations are of an autoerotic character and the sexual manifestations displayed by the child are the almost universal infantile masturbation which serves to prepare the genitals for their future functions; thumbsucking, according to many observers, connects directly or indirectly with autoerotic sexual activities.[10] I have studied a number of patients who retained this autoerotic sexual manifestation until late in life and I could definitely ascertain that it was a sexual activity pure and simple. In a number of cases thumbsucking continued until masturbation started and in a few cases both were practised synchronously. I know a young widow of thirty-five years who, in spite of all efforts to break herself of the habit, sucked her thumb until she married at twenty-five years and resumed it with the beginning of her widowhood. She told me she had no difficulty in stopping it soon after marriage, but that it returned a few weeks after her husband's death. The anus and the bladder outlets are also erogenous zones of infantile life, and neurotics often retain them in later life.* Thus Z., twenty years old, had an uncontrolable desire to withhold his urine. He stated that there was much pleasure in the discomfort and that that was the reason for repeating it. His mother told me that he wet the bed to the age of fifteen and that as a child he would remain on the chamber for hours before be could be made to move his bowels. The child at first knows no other sexual object except itself. It is only in the later stages of development that it goes over to the love object.

Besides the erogenous zones the child shows those components which are designated as partial impulses. Among these we have the impulse for looking and showing and for cruelty which manifest themselves somewhat independently of the erogenous zones and later enter into intimate relationship with the sexual life; but along with the erogenous sexual activity they are noticeable even in the infantile years as separate and independent strivings. In later life they are repressed and subjected to the primacy of the genitals which serve the functions of procreation. The energies emanating from them are then deflected from the sexual and directed to important social aims. This is the so-called process of *sublimation*. Thus, sublimation of the homosexual com-

* *Cf.* Chapter XI, on Anal Eroticism.

ponent gives origin to the psychic process of loathing and morality; the sublimation of the infantile looking and exhibitionism gives rise to shame, and the sublimation of the sadistic and masochistic components to disgust, pity and similar feelings. These reactions formed during the sexual latency period—from the fourth year to the beginning of puberty, eleven—make up the character of the person and later give us a good indication of his early sexual life. I regret that I am unable to discuss here more fully the sexual theories expounded by Freud; those who are interested in the subject should study his interesting and profound book, "The Three Contributions to the Sexual Theory." I will merely add that after carefully studying the sexual development in its relation to the normal neurotic individuals, Freud concluded that the constitutional sexual predisposition of the child is "polymorphous-perverse" and that from this constitution the so-called normal behavior of the sexual function results through a repression of certain components. The child has no conception of moral or esthetic feelings and it is only after the primitive impulses are repressed that the normal being evolves. By referring to the infantile character of sexuality the connection can be formed among the normal, perversions, and neuroses. The normal results through the repression of certain partial impulses and components of the infantile predisposition and through a subordination of the rest under the primacy of the genital zones. The perversions correspond to disturbances of this relationship due to a superior compulsive-like development of some of the partial impulses, while the neuroses can be traced to a marked repression of the libidinous strivings. However, it must be remembered that the symptoms do not by any means result at the expense only of the so-called normal sexual impulse (at least not exclusively or preponderately), but they represent the converted expression of impulses which might be designated as perverse if they could manifest themselves directly in phantasies and act without deviating from consciousness. The symptoms are therefore partially formed at the cost of abnormal sexuality. "The neurosis is, so to say, the negative of the perversion."[11]

Moreover, there is a congenital variation in the sexual constitution, the existence of which can naturally only be established through its later manifestations. It manifests itself in a preponderance of one or another of the manifold sources of the sexual feeling and it must always come to expression in the final result even if it should remain within normal limits. To be sure, certain variations of the original disposition even without further aid must necessarily lead to the formation of an abnormal sexual life. This may be called "degenerative" and considered as an expression of hereditary deterioration. In this connection Freud states that in more than half of the severe cases of hysteria, compulsion neuroses, etc., treated by him by psychotherapy he positively succeeded in demonstrating syphilis in their fathers before marriage. The patients showed absolutely no sign of hereditary lues, so that the abnormal sexual constitution was to be considered as the last off-shoot of the luetic heredity. In my own cases I found even less than a third in which syphilis could be demonstrated in parents.

If in the course of development certain strong components experience a repression the following result takes place: the sexual excitations are produced as usual, but are prevented from attaining their aim by psychic hindrances and are driven off into many other paths until they express themselves in symptoms. The sexual life of such persons begins like that of perverts. A considerable part of their childhood is filled up with perverse sexual activity which occasionally extends far beyond the period of maturity, but owing to inner reasons a repressive change results before or after puberty and henceforth there appears a neurosis instead of a perversion[12]; and confining ourselves for the present to hysteria it may be said that hysteria is the result of a conflict between the libido and the sexual repression and that the hysterical symptoms have the value of a compromise between both psychic streams. We must bear in mind that it is the mental conflict which is the essential causative factor and not the sexual moment as such. The resultant compromise of such conflict generally causes the sexual wishes to be consciously rejected and unconsciously accepted. The wish is then repressed, but the sum of excitement finds its way into bodily innervation and forms the hysterical symptom.

Let me cite an example.

A married woman of forty-nine years who suffered from hysteria for more than twenty-two years showed as one of her symptoms a very painful contracted and paralyzed right arm which had been so for more than three years. The muscles of the arm and shoulder region were completely anesthetic and deep needle pricks were not perceived, but the slightest attempt to straighten out the member was most painful. Indeed the pain was the chief symptom. It would be impossible for me to give here the full analysis of the symptom. I will merely mention some of the psychic constellations.

Due to a number of sexual traumas sustained in childhood all sexual feelings were repressed and, as a result, she was totally frigid when she was married. Indeed coitus was both painful and disgusting to her. This produced marked marital unhappiness, her husband failed to understand her condition, and what made matters worse was the fact that he found her masturbating in her sleep. When he first noticed it he was very indignant and tried to call her to account for it, but she continued to sleep; he tried to arouse her, but she did not respond. He thought at first that she was shamming, but finally concluded that "she had a fit" and reported the matter to the family physician. This somnambulistic state during which she masturbated was repeated on an average of five to six times a week. There was complete amnesia for this action. She at first refused to believe it, but she was finally convinced of it by her own sister, who saw her do it on the occasion of sleeping with her. She then sought the aid of a physician who gave her large doses of bromide and advised her to wear a sock over her hand and firmly tie her arm in complete flexion While she was being treated for her masturbation it was reported to her that her husband carried on some illicit relations with one of the girls she employed. She absolutely refused to believe this, and no amount of urging on the part of her husband's own relatives could induce her to dismiss this girl. This girl was the daughter of a very poor woman and it was out of compassion that she took her into her millinery establishment and taught her the profession. This state of affairs continued for months. She was extremely jealous, yet her pride would not allow her to take any action in the matter. It was after a quarrel about some other matters, during which her husband grasped her by the right arm that it became painful and developed into the condition noted above. As she was the moving spirit in the millinery establishment the business had to be given up, as she was totally incapacitated by her malady.

Here we see the conflict was between the libido and the repression. The repressed sexual feelings made her consciously frigid, but unconsciously passionate. When her masturbation was brought to her consciousness she took all the precautions to prevent it, but as usual she was unsuccessful. Her husband's faithlessness gave rise to another conflict. Her pride gained the upper hand and she absolutely refused to believe what everyone else saw and what she herself could not fail to see. When her husband grasped her by this arm, which was the cause of so much mental pain—it was the one with which she masturbated—the conversion took place. The symptom, as Freud puts it, was the result of a compromise between two opposing affects, one of which strove to bring to a realization a partial impulse or a component of the sexual constitution, while the other strove to suppress the same.[13] This symptom, as we see, served a double purpose. It stopped the masturbation and incapacitated her to such an extent that the business had to be given up and the girl who caused her so many pangs had to go. The pain was also the punishment for the underlying sexual desire. She never masturbated with her left hand, nor has she ever been seen masturbating since she was cured by psychanalysis.

In analyzing neurotic symptoms Freud found that the dream played a great part in the individual's life. This gave origin to the epoch-making book, "The Interpretation of Dreams."* The dream is not at all absurd and senseless, but has a definite meaning when analyzed, and in the experienced hand it is the most valuable instrument for penetrating the mind. In the neurotic patient the subject of the dream generally refers to the origin of the neurosis, *i.e.*, to the repressed material, but due to the many distortions and transformations only few and

* Translated by A. A. Brill. George Allen, London, and the Macmillan Co., New York.

hidden associations show allusions to the repressed experience. Psychanalysis explains the different components of the dream and thus reveals the repressed ideas which are at the basis of the neurosis. The dream is divided into the manifest and latent thoughts. The former are remembered by the dreamer on awakening, while the latter represent the thoughts of the dream before they were subjected to the distortion. When the translation is complete we find that the latent thoughts of the dream contain the fulfilment of a repressed wish.[14] The same holds true in the psychoneurotic symptoms. In the words of Freud, "The hysterical symptom, like all other psychic formations, is the expression of a wish fulfilment."[15]

In the same way the repression continues to evince itself in normal conscious life; in other words, the wish fulfilment normally manifests itself during the waking state just as it does in the dream and in the neurotic symptoms. This can be readily seen if we analyze the abnormal or the so-called accidental actions of every-day life. In his very interesting and instructive book, "The Psychopathology of Every Day Life,"[16] Freud shows that mere lapses of memory, speech and writing, as well as the common mistakes are not at all accidental, but when analyzed have a reason. Thus the forgetting of a name which we have once known implies that either directly or indirectly there is something painful or disagreeable connected with it. A mistake in talking is usually what the speaker really means. In other words, the repression influences our waking state just as it does the dream and the psychoneurotic symptoms. Just as the latent thought of the dream, the psychoneurotic symptom represents a fulfilled wish and both the dream and the neurosis seem incomprehensible until explained by psychanalysis.

I will now cite a brief analysis of an obsession. One of my patients a young man twenty-six years old, suffered from a typical compulsion neurosis, the main symptom being an obsessive action which consisted in a rapid upward movement of his arms, as though holding back or pushing up something. This action became very annoying to him and his family. He was often compelled to do it in public and it interfered with his work as a diamond cutter. Before proceeding with the analysis I will mention something concerning the technique.

On analyzing psychoneurotic symptoms the patient is required to lie on his back on a lounge and the physician sits behind the patient's head at the head of the lounge. The object of this position is to avoid all muscular exertion and distraction, thus allowing a thorough concentration of attention on the patient's own psychic activities. In my experience the same purpose can be accomplished with the patient sitting in front of you in a comfortable chair. We then ask the patient to tell all he knows of the symptom and we usually find a number of memory gaps. These he is urged to fill in by concentration of attention on the subject and by repeating all thoughts originating in this connection. Before proceeding we must have the patient's promise that he will frankly repeat to us all the thoughts occurring to him in the order of their sequence, even thoughts that are painful or embarrassing. This is Freud's method of free association. We are also alive to the fact that the psychoneurotic symptom is often a symbolic expression of the original repressed thoughts and we therefore resort to Freud's method of interpretation, that is we look for symbolic expressions, psychopathological actions and make use of the analysis of dreams. For unless one has mastered the triad of Freud's psychology, "The Three Contributions to the Sexual Theory," "The Psychopathology of Every Day Life" and "The Interpretation of Dreams," he is unable to use or judge Freud's psychanalytic method. With this digression we will now return to our patient.

On being questioned concerning his obsessive action it was found that it concealed the obsessive thought "God may get into me." This thought obsessed him for months, and realizing the absurdity of it, he was ashamed to tell it to anybody. This was then followed by the obsessive action described above which was a protective mechanism against the thought and signified "I will pull Him out again." As the word "God" seemed to be the most important word in the obsession I asked him to concentrate his mind on this word and tell me all the associations it recalled to him. He gave the following: "God—father—I am always bothered by the foolish thought that God will get into me." He suddenly stopped and on being urged to continue he said that something just occurred to him which had nothing to do with the thought of God and which he would not like to tell unless it was absolutely necessary. On being told to continue he stated that it recalled to him that about six months ago while being at work a fellow workingman once asked him to look out of the window and when he did so he saw two dogs in the act of copulation. This was very embarrassing to him. He turned his eyes away from the scene, but he could not banish a number of fancies which then came to his mind. One thought was "How would it be to get into the dog?" He soon repressed these thoughts and kept on repeating to himself "I will not get into the dog, the dog may get into me." Now if the word dog is read backward you will find that it spells God and gives the key to the whole obsession. For years this patient was in the habit of turning words about. He showed me a diary which was filled with mirror writing which he used because he did not want anyone in the house to know his affairs. We note that he at first consciously changed the idea "to get into the dog" into "the dog may get into me" and as the idea was disagreeable it was repressed and the word "dog" was then unconsciously changed into God. This completed the obsession.*

As will be shown later the same mechanisms are found in the dream, in the neologisms of the insane and in the normal. I am sure that the majority of my readers are aware of the fact that the Sesrun Club is the nurses' club and perhaps few know that the Yvel Jewelry company is the Levy Jewelry company. The basis of each cryptogram is a painful idea. Nurses' Club neither looks nor sounds as dignified as Sesrun Club, which may pass as a millionaires' organization, and the Yvel Jewelry company looks better and is perhaps more profitable than would be the Levy Jewelry company.

This is a very simple example of the psychanalysis of an obsession, perhaps too simple to impress some of you with the gravity of the work, but we cannot change the workings of the mind. Those who analyze psychoneurotic symptoms and the utterances of the insane can always find such mechanisms. Do not, however, think that the analyses of this obsession and the afore-described hysterical paralysis were as simple as I presented them. I merely give you the result obtained after weeks and months of painstaking work. It would have been impossible to give here the full analysis of any of the cases, as an entire volume would be required for a detailed account of any one. Indeed, psychanalysis takes time; the treatment of a chronic case usually takes from six months to a few years, but the most refractory chronic cases have been cured by this treatment. Both cases mentioned

* For detailed description of compulsion neurosis see Chapter IV.

were cured by psychanalysis after everything else was tried in vain.

Lest there should be some misunderstanding about the facility of the psychanalytic treatment and in order to demonstrate how we actually work I shall next confine myself to the discussion of the theory of dreams.

References

1. Freud: Selected Papers on Hysteria and Other Psychoneuroses, p. 2, Trans. by A. A. Brill, Monograph Series Mental and Nervous Dis. Pub. Co. 2d Ed.

2. *L. c.*, p. 5.

3. Freud: Ueber Psychoanalyse, Deuticke, Wien, 1910.

4. Freud: Selected Papers, p. 87.

5. Freud: *L. c.*, p. 125.

6. *L. c.*, p. 126.

7. *Cf.* Chap. V.

8. Selected Papers, p. 188.

9. Freud: Three Contributions to the Sexual Theory, p. 38. Trans. by A. A. Brill, Monograph Series.

10. *Cf.* Holt, Diseases of Infancy and Childhood, p. 739, Second Edition.

11. Freud: *L. c.*, p. 27. See also Chapter IV.

12. Freud: *L. c.*

13. Selected Papers, p. 198.

14. *Cf.* Chap. II.

15. Freud: *L. c.*, 197.

16. English translation in preparation, *Cf.* also Chap. VII.

CHAPTER II

DREAMS

Their Structure and Mechanism, Technique of Interpretation, Symbolism and their Relation to the Neuroses and Psychoses

"*Der müde Gebundene der in Fesseln liegt kann nicht erwachen, der müde Gebundene träumt von Freiheit.*"—*Hauptmann.*

From time immemorial the dream has been the subject of much interest and speculation. Since the early Greek period numerous theories have been propounded and entertained in the realms of religion and of science, but not until within recent years has investigation of the dream proceeded on a true psychological basis. It would be superfluous and quite impossible to review here the many curious theories held at different epochs in the world's history concerning the dream; suffice it to say that ancients and moderns differ very little in their views. The ancient Greeks believed that the dream was an inspiration of the gods, that it was simply a warning or prophecy of things to come and they always gave credence to it. Kindred thoughts are expressed in the Bible. Joseph interpreted all dreams as a foreboding of the future, "what God is about to do he showeth unto Pharoah;" and as the Scriptures inform us steps were immediately taken to prepare for the approaching famine. These views have come down to us traditionally and disregarding here the numerous scientific and pseudoscientific theories, we may say that the present popular belief in dreams differs in no wise from that of the classical Greeks and the ancient Egyptians. Every race and religion still looks upon the dream as something supernatural and objective, as an inspiration coming from above; and the laity still continues to believe in its reality. The gambler dreams his horses or lottery numbers, the Indian medicine man dreams his remedies, and not seldom we hear even of "dreams coming true."

Modern psychology has continued the work of ancient writers and as a result we have numerous valuable contributions to the problem of the dream; numerous attempts have been made to show the relation of the dream to normal and abnormal life,[1] but so far as I know no author has solved the problem of the dream so ingeniously and successfully as Professor Freud.[2] As mentioned previously in developing his psychology of the psychoneuroses Freud found that the dream plays a very important part in the psyche of the individual. The dream is not a senseless jumble, but a perfect mechanism and when analyzed it is found to contain the fulfilment of a wish; it always treats of the inmost thoughts of personality and for that reason gives us the best access to the unconscious. No psychanalysis is complete, nay possible, without the analysis of dreams. The dream not only helps us to interpret symptoms, but is often an invaluable instrument in diagnosis and treatment. The causative factors of many neuroses are extremely vague and usually unconscious to the patient, and it is by means of the dream that the underlying etiological factors are disclosed.

In order to understand the mechanism of dreams it will be necessary to bear in mind Freud's conception of repression.[3] To forget is a part of human nature; this is so obvious that we never even stop to think about it. Yet when we examine the things forgotten we soon find that there is a method in forgetting; our forgetting seems to follow a kind of selection. It was Freud who first called attention to the motives of forgetting. If we exclude organic brain disturbances, we find that we are most apt to forget painful or disagreeable impressions. This forgetting, as everyone knows, is purposeful and desired. The individual strives at all times to rid himself of the unbearable either by settling the situation in question when possible or by directly crowding it out of his mind. When we meet with mishaps or failures to which we cannot adequately react, we grieve over them for a time and then make desperate efforts to forget them —that is, we repress them. Moreover, the phantasies which are common to both normal and abnormal persons may be of a disagreeable nature or present an unattainable object and may therefore be repressed. It often happens that such phantasies are repressed before they are really grasped by full consciousness. The repressed material, or, in the language of Jung, the complexes are pushed into the unconscious and there they remain in a dormant state.[4] Now and then they are recalled by some association, but like disturbed ghosts they soon return to their resting place. Jung has shown likewise that they can be artificially evoked and in this country this has been corroborated by many observers. The repression is not, however, always successful and as I shall show later a splitting of consciousness may result. The repressed complexes then strive for manifestation and the resultant psychic conflict may produce a psychosis or neurosis. In brief, both normal and neurotic individuals possess a certain amount of repression. In the former this usually remains inert, manifesting itself only now and then in psychopathological actions[5] or dreams, while in the latter it forms in addition the symptoms of the neurosis or psychosis.[6] But no matter in what form the repression comes to the surface—whether in the form of dreams, in psychoneurotic symptoms, or in the utterances or manifestations of the insane—it is always so distorted as to be unrecognizable to the individual.

What causes this distortion? When we examine the literature of the past and present we observe that writers frequently resort to all sorts of detours, euphemisms and symbolisms when they wish to express something which would sound either harsh or objectionable to polite society. Thus we find that the words "thigh" and "staff" are often used in the Bible to express that part which represents the male* and nowadays journalism makes use of exactly the same devices. Witness the cartoons and jokes in the daily papers.[7] We all know that many of the jokes of our best comedians would be considered extremely offensive if direct expression were given to the underlying thoughts. The reason why such mechanisms are necessary is quite obvious. It is the fear of the censor. We

* See Genesis xxiv, 2, and xlvii, 29; Hebrews xi, 21,

all know what would happen to the comedian who, instead of uttering some innocent quibble as "Willie Rose rose because he sat on a pin" would venture to give the bare underlying thought. This censor has been established by society for its own protection and the stricter the censor the more concealed and funnier are the means of representation. In the same way the distortions in the dream and in psychotic symptoms are the work of the psychic censor. This, too, is a protective mechanism for the good of the organism.

The formation of dreams is brought about by the working of the two psychic forces (streams or systems), one of which forms the wish of the dream, while the other exerts its censorship on this wish and thus produces the distortion. The reason for our belief in this second psychic force possessing the power of censoring is as follows: The latent thoughts of the dream are not known until the dream has been subjected to analysis. What we remember on awakening are the manifest contents of the dream emanating from the former. We can therefore assume that the admission to consciousness is the prerogative of the second psychic system. Nothing from the first system can reach consciousness without having passed through the second system, and the latter allows nothing to pass without exercising its prerogative of censoring. At the point of transition between the two systems we have the psychic censor, which after exercising its function allows to pass only that which is agreeable to it and restrains everything else. Whatever is rejected by the censor is in a state of repression. As will be shown this psychic censor is nothing but the inhibitions formed throughout our whole life by our religious and ethical training.

As mentioned before the dream is divided into the manifest and the latent dream contents. The former comprise all the delusive sensory impressions which are recalled by the dreamer on awakening; while the latter comprise the fundamental thoughts of the dream as they existed before being subjected to the distortion of the psychic censor. The manifest content of the dream seems absurd and incoherent, but by psychanalysis it can readily be translated into the latent thoughts, which always show the fulfilment of a wish.

When we watch the development of a human being especially during the first few years of its existence, we are particularly impressed with one fact, to wit: that the child is insatiable in its desires. As soon as the child sees the light of this world it makes known its wants and as soon as it grows older they become proportionately greater. At first these desires are purely primitive, but with advancing age they become more complicated. Thus a child of a few days old cries when hungry or uncomfortable, while at a later age it may cry because it is not rocked to sleep or because it is not allowed to suck its thumb. Here we no longer deal with necessary wants, but with pleasurable desires; for the child could fall asleep without being rocked and should get along without thumbsucking. When we observe a child at about the age of two, or at an older age, we can clearly see that it is a constant pleasure seeker. All its activities are directed toward the realization of both necessary and pleasurable desires, especially the latter, and the older the child becomes the more it wants. It would be no exaggeration to assume that if this condition were allowed to continue, the whole world would be too small to supply the wants of a single individual. This idea is very well expressed in a pretty fable which I had read years ago, I believe in Socin's Arabic Grammar. The story tells that Alexander of Macedon, while traveling after his numerous victories, one day came unexpectedly to a strange place. He wanted to enter, but the door was locked. He knocked on the door and asked to be admitted. After being ignored for some time he was finally told that he was at the door of Paradise and that no mortal could enter there. "But I am Alexander the Great," he remonstrated. "At least give me some memento that I may be able to say I was here." A hand was extended through the door and gave him a human eye. Alexander was chagrined and baffled. He could not understand the significance of the souvenir. In his distress he appealed to the wise men of his entourage and after considerable study and rumination one of these—the wisest of them all—undertook to solve the riddle. He ordered that a scale be brought and he placed the eye upon one side of it. He placed Alexander's jewels upon the other. The eye was heavier. More gold and jewels were placed on the other side, but the eye still outweighed the valuables. To the surprise and consternation of Alexander the Great no amount of precious stones or gold was heavy enough to counterbalance the eye. The scale containing it bore down steadily. The wise man thereupon covered the eye with some earth and, behold! the scales turned. The eye balanced no more than its actual weight. The explanation by the wise man was as follows: the eye uncovered signifies the living eye, the covered eye signifies one dead. While man lives he is insatiable; the more the eye sees the more it desires. Once it is covered with earth it has no need of anything. This souvenir was therefore intended as a rebuke to Alexander's unbridled ambition. That this moral lesson left little impression on the insatiable conqueror is shown by the fact that he died of his insane excesses at the early age of thirty-two years.

To-day there are no more worlds to conquer, but we are all Alexanders, none the less. Each of us who is not afflicted with the emotional deterioration of the Schizophrenic is dominated by ambitions and is never perfectly contented. And were it not for the severe checking the individual constantly experiences from the very beginning of his childhood, which causes him to give up most of his desires, it would be impossible to live in any society, savage or enlightened.

This inhibiting process begins in childhood and is continued throughout life. Thus a child of fifteen months cries for a bird kept by her parents as a pet. She is not satisfied with merely looking at it and hearing it sing, but she wants to touch and handle it. As this would be detrimental to the well being of the bird she is made to forego this pleasure in spite of her bitter crying. A little girl of four years wants toys belonging to other children. She is very unhappy and irritable because she cannot get them, but with her mother's help, she finally abandons this desire. At an earlier age this same child unceremoniously appropriated other children's toys and it was only after being punished that she desisted from this highway robbery and developed the sense of property. So, throughout the whole course of our existence, society (religion and ethics) teaches us to curb our desires and to give up what we want. We want much and we get comparatively little, but *we never stop wanting.*

When we try to examine how children learn to give up their desires we are soon struck by the fact that they never really give up anything entirely. A girl of four years after being told by her mother that she cannot get a certain toy which she saw in the hand of another child, brooded over it for awhile and then drew on the sidewalk with chalk what she thought was a picture of this toy and played with it as though it were the real toy. The little girl of fifteen months forgets the bird and is always appeased when she gets a wooden bird or a picture book of birds. You all know how boys ride on sticks for want of horses and that nearly all the games played by children represent unattainable desires. Nor do we see those actions only in early life when the child cannot differentiate between fiction and reality. If we continue to observe we find that these same children as they grow older and know that a stick is not a horse and that a drawing of a toy is not a real toy, nevertheless still attain what they want. Thus a little boy goes to the Zoological garden where he sees tigers. He remarks that he would like to have a few tigers. His father laughs at him and points out that he would have no room for them if he had them. The boy then dreams that he had five little tigers in a bird cage hanging in his room. All this goes to show that the human mind possesses the faculty of overcoming difficulties and attains its desires in spite of the obstacles raised by nature and society. This is Prof. Freud's theory of wish fulfilment. In brief this theory states that whatever is denied us in reality we can nevertheless realize in some other way. In his sleep the poor man has much money, the prisoner his freedom; the lame man runs races, and the ambitious man sees himself at the goal of his ambition. In other words, the dream represents the realization of a wish; its motive is a wish.

In this respect dreams are divided into three classes: 1. Those which represent an unrepressed wish as fulfilled, as seen in the so-called convenience dream and in children's dreams. For example, we often dream of enjoying cold fresh water after a supper of sardines, olives or other salty food. The thirst incites the dream which tries to appease the sleeper so as to avoid disturbance of sleep. A boy of five dreams of finding pennies and nickels and on awakening expresses his disappointment by crying for his money. A little girl of four dreams of chocolate almonds and on awakening insists that someone has taken her "big box of chocolate almonds." 2. Those which represent the realization of a repressed wish in an entirely concealed form, examples of which I shall give later. 3. Those which represent the realization of a repressed wish in a form insufficiently or only partially concealed. The last group of dreams is generally accompanied by fear, which interrupts the dream and which takes the place of the distortion found in the second group. Dreams accompanied by fear are of a sexual nature; the ideation causing the fear in the dream was once a wish which was later subjected to repression.[8] There are some dreams of a painful nature which are not, however, perceived as such by the dreamer. These merely show the insignificance and lack of psychic validity of the dream. In these cases analysis always shows that we deal with the hidden fulfilment of a repressed wish. Thus, one of my patients dreamed that she saw her oldest boy laid out in a casket, and yet she was totally unconcerned about it. Having been told previously that a dream represents the fulfilment of a wish she now insisted that this theory must be wrong, as she would never entertain any such wish regarding her boy. Psychanalysis, however, revealed the following facts: her husband had died and left her with two children; she had then married a widower with two children. They are very happy, but as they already have four children they cannot afford to rear any more. She has frequently expressed the wish "to have an offspring as the result of her second marriage, as it would strengthen the union, but having four children in the family, this is out of the question." The dream fulfils her wish by showing her that there are only three children in the family. A man of thirty dreamed that he saw his brother's head split open and bleeding and was not at all worried about it. He, too, objected to the theory of wish fulfilment. Analysis showed that he referred to his brother M., a boy of sixteen years, whom he had thought incorrigible. He had read recently an article in a Sunday newspaper saying that bad boys could be cured by trephining the skull and exposing the brain—which at once caused him to think of his brother. The dream realized his wish by showing him his brother with his brain exposed.

Recently a patient came to me and disputed the theory

of wish fulfilment. To prove his assertion he stated that the night before he had dreamed that he had syphilis. I could readily prove that the dream showed the realization of a wish. This patient was being treated by me for psychosexual impotence and the day before his dream we discussed promiscuous sexuality. I called his attention to the dangers of infection and spoke about proper precautions, etc. He grimly remarked "There is no danger of my becoming infected. I couldn't if I tried." The dream realizes his wish that he can become infected; meaning that he is no longer sexually impotent.

Still another patient suffering from the same disease dreamed that he was bald. He too objected to the theory of wish realization inasmuch as he is only thirty-five years old and he surely would not like to be bald. I told him that except with children a dream should never be judged by the manifest content. When he began to give "free associations" to the dream he suddenly thought of a smutty joke which he was unwilling to reproduce. I insisted that he should tell me everything, otherwise the analysis would have to be dropped. The joke is credited to one of our witty statesmen and tells how at a social gathering a young lady heard this statesman use the word "eunuch." Not knowing the meaning of the word she turned to the statesman and said "Mr. X—, I heard you use the word 'eunuch.' What is a eunuch?" The statesman was embarrassed and hesitatingly answered "A eunuch is a balled (bald) man." The young lady looked at his head and said "Then you are a eunuch." "Oh, no," he replied, "I am too bald (two balled)." My patient heard this joke the day before the dream and he laughed very heartily over it, but his loud and prolonged laughter was only hiding his inner pain, for this smutty joke brought to mind his own complex; he was a eunuch himself. The dream was, therefore, a reaction to his mental pain and showed him that he was not a eunuch. He is too bald (two balled) like the statesman in the story. The other determinants are the identification of the bald head with the head of the penis, an identification which I have repeatedly observed in dreams and psychoses. One of my patients, a young præcox, had one mannerism which was shown by a constant rubbing of the top of the head. After doing this for a few months he had a good-sized tonsure which was rapidly increasing. I could definitely ascertain that the patient went through a form of masturbation. He was not allowed to masturbate his penis so he used his head. Another determinant for the baldness in the dream is the fact that, like sexual impotence, baldness, too, is considered as a sign of physical weakness and senile decay. These examples show that even dreams which are, in the manifest content, the opposite of wishes, nevertheless contain a wish when we find the latent content.

The transformation of the latent into the manifest content of the dream is effected as follows by the so-called "dream work" (Traumarbeit). During our waking state a number of thought structures are constantly being formed. This activity is never finished during the day, and the sum of energy required for the production of these thoughts would be sufficient to hold the interest of the individual to such an extent as to interfere with sleep. These day remnants are, therefore, changed into dreams by the dream work and the elements threatening disturbance of sleep are thus removed. *The dream is therefore the guardian of sleep.* But in order that the work of the dream may act the day remnants must be capable of wish formation, for it is the wish that forms the nucleus of the dream.

When we compare the latent thoughts of the dream with its manifest content we find that the former is perfectly comprehensible as soon as we discover it, while the latter is usually incomprehensible and absurd and comparable to hieroglyphics or a rebus. We are also struck by the marked *condensation,* which takes place in the transformation of the thought into the content of the dream.* The manifest dream when written may fill a few lines, while the analysis containing the thoughts underlying the dream usually fills many pages. This condensation is effected by the omission and the subsequent compression of syllables, words, pictures or situations which have been present in the thoughts underlying the dream. This accounts for the many gaps, absurdities and neologisms in the manifest content of the dream. Thus, one of my German patients saw a monkey in his dream, and by freely associating to the word "monkey" we got monkey—chimpanzee—Schimpfen Sie McKenzie (which may be translated here by "Give it to him, McKenzie"). This recalled a quarrel between two laborers, McKenzie and X. the day before the dream. The patient actually heard this very exclamation, "Give it to him, McKenzie," and as a diligent student of English he immediately translated it into the above German sentence.

*Condensation is a fusion of events, pictures and elements of speech.

This is further determined by the fact that the features of the pugnacious McKenzie made him think of a monkey and that the quarrel took place near a zoological garden. It is through this process of condensation that the manifest thoughts of the dream are "overdetermined." The individual thoughts of the dream are not only represented in the dream by many elements, but the elements of the dream are manifoldly determined by the thoughts of the dream. In the analysis of dreams one often finds all kinds of composites such as composite pictures and collective personalities, all of which are produced by this process of condensation.

Another effect of the dream work is brought about by the process of *displacement.* Thus the elements which seem most conspicuous in the content of the dream do not necessarily have corresponding importance in the thoughts of the dream. An insignificant element may represent the main thought and *vice versa,* events, thoughts, sentences, words and pictures may be turned around. By the process of overdetermination the psychic validity of the main element may be displaced or transferred to some triviality. The same process is met in the obsessions of neurotics.[9] The formation of the dream is chiefly due to these two processes of displacement and condensation.

Besides the processes of condensation and displacement which we have found so effective in the transformation of the latent into the manifest thoughts we must take into account two other factors, viz., the manner of representation and the secondary elaboration, to which I shall only allude. There is no intellectual activity in the dream. What in the manifest content impresses us as a process of reasoning or judgment is not due to the work of the dream, but has reached the manifest content from the thoughts of the dream to which it properly belonged. Logical relationships are not represented in the dream. The dream makes use of visual pictures which are reproduced by similarity, identification and symbolization. The affects are not influenced by the dream work though they are very often displaced. The dream also omits all the "ifs" and "buts" and whatever may be in the subjunctive mood in our waking state is transferred into the indicative present in the dream. This accounts for the fact that in the dream the blind see, the lame run and the poor are wealthy. The "If I were" is changed in the dream into "I am."

To illustrate the relation of the dream to the neurosis I shall cite the following case:

Case: Miss G., twenty-eight years old, American, came to me in January, 1908, because she had been "very nervous" for about three months. Her family history showed that her father died of nephritis and had a "stroke" (left hemiplegia) a few months before he died. She had been well until three months before. Since then she had suffered from insomnia, irritability, loss of appetite, constipation, headache, uncalled for worry, crying spells and anxious expectation. Her mother stated that she had entirely changed, that she expressed pessimistic ideas, often repeating that she would like to die. Examination showed all the symptoms enumerated. The patient was pretty, she showed no stigmata and was above the average in intelligence. While reciting her story she showed the typical *belle indifférence* often found in hysteria. She smiled when I asked her why she felt so depressed and could give no reason for it. She knew that she really had nothing to worry about and that she had everything to live for, yet she could not "shake off the blue feeling." One of the most distressing thoughts was that something might happen to her mother.

To those acquainted with the language of hysteria this means just the opposite. It was merely a reaction of the wish that she might lose her mother, and, as we shall see later, there was a reason for that wish. Physically there was nothing worth mentioning. I diagnosticated the case as a mild anxiety hysteria[10] with imperfect conversion.

I saw her a number of times, but made no progress in the treatment. To my question she always answered "I feel about the same." I then thought of psychanalysis and with that in view I asked her to write out her dreams and bring them to me. She was sure that she never dreamed except when her stomach was out of order, but promised to comply with my request if ever she should and one day brought me the following dream:

"*I dreamed that I was in a lonely country place and was anxious to reach my home in Liconow or Liconor Bay, but could not get there. Every time I made a move there was a wall in the way. It looked like a street full of walls. My legs were as heavy as lead. I could only walk very slowly as if I were very weak or very old. Then there was a flock of chickens, but that seemed to be in a crowded city street, and they—the chickens—ran after me and the biggest of all said something like "Come with me into the dark.*"

This dream seems absurd enough and as the dreamer remarked, "It is so ridiculous that I am ashamed to tell it. Whoever heard of such a thing as chickens talking?" She was assured that it must mean something and the analysis proceeded.

It would be too long and immaterial for the purposes of this work to give here the whole analysis which, when recorded, covered over eight pages of foolscap. Only the principal associations and symbolic expressions necessary to explain the dream will be enumerated.

On asking the dreamer what the most vivid part of the dream was she answered that it was the second part relating to the chickens. When asked to repeat the thoughts evoked by concentrating her mind on the word "chickens" she gave the following: "I could only see the biggest chicken, all the others seemed blurred; it was unusually big and had a very long neck and it spoke to me—the street recalls where I used to go to school—I graduated from public school when I was thirteen—the block was always crowded with children from school"—she then began to blush and laugh and when asked to explain her actions said: "It recalls the happy school days when I was young and had no worries—I even had a beau, a pupil from the male department. There was a male and a female department in the same school and most of my girl friends had beaux—we used to meet after school hours and walk home together. My beau's name was F. He was lanky and thin and the girls used to tease me about him. Whenever they saw him coming they said, 'Belle, here comes your chicken'—that was his nickname among the boys." On being asked if she now understood who the chicken in the dream was she laughingly said: "You don't mean to say that the chicken with the long neck was Mr. F.?" When asked if she still kept up her acquaintance with Mr. F. she stated that she had not seen him for the last few months, but prior to that she saw him quite often. On further analysis it was found that this early schoolday love was still kept up. He had proposed to her no less than three times, but she had never given him any definite answer. She only "liked" him and her family opposed him on account of his financial position. The last time she met him was at a military ball. He was an officer of a military organization and "he looked quite handsome in his smart uniform." He danced with her and "was very kind," but he did not propose. She frankly admitted that she looked for a fourth proposal at this ball and that she was quite ready to accept him. She had heard only recently that he was paying attention to another young lady, a thing which caused her considerable annoyance—to put it in her own words, "I can only blame myself and I will have to forget it."

We see that the most impossible and ludicrous part of the dream, that is, "the talking of the chicken," is now quite plain. The "chicken" is simply the nickname of Mr. F., who is the hero of the dream. There were other chickens, but they were blurred, that is, there were other young suitors, but they were relegated to the background.

The chicken said "*Come with me into the dark.*" The word "dark" evoked the following associations: indistinct—obscure—mystery—marriage. She recalled that after her father's death her mother once spoke sympathetically of Mr. F. saying "Money is not all," and philosophized on marriage in the following remarks: "You will never know a man until you have eaten a peck of salt with him" and "Marriage is a mystery." These words made a deep impression on her and the last Biblical quotation frequently recurred to her. We then see that in her mind the word "dark" was used synonomously with mystery and marriage, and hence we can understand its meaning in the chicken's speech. Briefly stated it was the fourth proposal of Mr. F.

The first part of the dream reads, "*I was in a lonely country place, etc.* "She stated that she recalled the beautiful country around H. Bay where she had been the preceding summer. She could not quite understand what Liconow or Liconor Bay meant and gave the following associations: Liconow—Lucknow—meaning a painting representing the famous battle of Lucknow which she had recently seen. The soldiers recalled the military organization at whose ball she had met Mr. F. The word "Liconor" suggested by sound association Lucarno and Lugano, two places which she had visited while abroad two years before. H. Bay often recalled the beautiful Italian lakes, Lucarno and Lugano, whither she hoped to go on her honeymoon. Finally, Liconor Bay resolved itself into LIK-ONOR BAY which, by sound association, can be readily recognized as "like, honor and obey." If "like" is substituted by "love" it gives the familiar formula well known to all maidens seriously contemplating matrimony. The dreamer used "like," because, as aforesaid, she thought she only "liked." Such condensations of words and ideas are not at all rare in dreams.

If we now rewrite the first sentence it will read as follows: "I was in a lonely country place and was anxious to reach my home in 'LIKe (love), hONOR, and oBEY,'" that is, "I was lonely and anxious to get married."

The next sentence reads "*But could not, etc.*" She stated that her legs "were as heavy as lead," she was alone and was afraid that something might happen, but she was unable to make any headway. The sensation of inhibition experienced in dreams, like the inability to make any headway when one most desires to do so, signifies a marked mental conflict. Here, too, it merely shows the great mental conflict in our dreamer's mind. She is anxious to marry. She "likes" Mr. F. Moreover, she is of an advanced age and, as the dream shows, she could walk only very slowly as if "she were weak or very old," that is, the difficulties on the road to matrimony increase with advancing age; she is weak and old, that is, she is an "old maid," an expression by which she often jocosely referred to herself in her waking state; all of these arguments are in favor of accepting Mr. F., but then her family is opposed to him. He is a nice enough young man, but he is unable to care for her in a manner befitting her station in life.

The dream continues: "*Every time I made a move there was a wall in the way, it looked like a street full of walls, etc.*" A street full of walls signifies Wall street, hence money—that was the real obstacle. When told of the interpretation she laughingly remarked "That's it exactly. I even thought very seriously of helping him along, as Pa left me some money, but then everything is invested in Wall street and there is a tacit understanding among ourselves that the whole estate shall be left intact until mother's death."

We now understand the latent thoughts of the dream. The first part can be translated as follows: I am twenty-eight years old, an old maid, and I am anxious to marry Mr. F., but then he is not rich enough to take care of me. I perhaps can help him financially. In the second part we find the wish realization, as here Mr. F. actually proposes to her for the fourth time.

These were the actual thoughts which had occupied our dreamer's mind for the past months and which, as she quite frankly admitted, she tried hard to forget. It is quite obvious that the dream deals here with the thoughts which a young lady would not consciously disclose even to her physician, and we can also understand why she was "ashamed to tell it" because she understood it unconsciously, though not consciously. The dream never deals with trivialities, and, no matter how simple and innocent it may seem, the analysis invariably shows that the thoughts behind it belong to the inmost recesses of personality. This accounts for the many resistances encountered during the analysis. The psychic censor constantly inhibits the painful or disagreeable complexes from becoming conscious and is also responsible for the rapid forgetting of dreams on awakening.

Dreams often help us to make a correct diagnosis. This is especially true in the anxiety states and homosexuality. People who are subject to nightmares or who have anxiety dreams usually suffer from lack of sexual gratification. I do not mean merely the gross sexual, but I use the word in the Freudian sense. We must be very careful in our examination, otherwise we may make mistakes. Thus a married woman suffered from a pronounced anxiety hysteria and was subject to frequent nightmares, but on being questioned she stated that her sexual life was normal. A few weeks later I discovered that she was suffering from frigidity and although she was married six years she never experienced an orgasm or any pleasure in coitus.

I have made many diagnoses of homosexuality from the patient's dreams. Many homosexuals go to doctors, but do not tell them the true state of affairs. They are usually sensitive and not knowing how the physician will look upon them they complain of something else. Thus, a homosexual whom I saw in the Vanderbilt clinic complained of pain in the thigh. His dream told me the true story. It also happens that the patients do not know that they are homosexual. This is usually the case with women, but I have seen at least two men who were ignorant of their being homosexual. Their dreams first called my attention to the fact. But it should be remembered that one is not to judge by the manifest content of the dream as does Näcke,[11] for a dream may not show anything of the gross homosexual in its manifest content and still be a homosexual dream. This is shown by the following dream brought to me by a man of thirty-five years: "*I saw two men. One looked at an open newspaper and the other watched him sidewise, reading his thoughts like a detective. Suddenly the latter stabbed the man with the newspaper by plunging a dagger into his heart. Great commotion—crowd.*"

After reading the dream as it was written by the patient immediately on awakening three hours before, I asked him to tell me the dream from memory. He reproduced the dream correctly, but made one mistake; instead of saying that the dagger was plunged into the heart he said that it was plunged into the back. My object in asking him to reproduce the dream was this: From the association experiments of the Zurich school[12] we know that a failure of reproduction is a complex indicator; that is, whenever the answer is forgotten it shows that the word or passage in question is of marked emotional accentuation and contains something cryptic. It has the same mechanism as the lapsus linguæ or any other mistake. Now let us take up the analysis: A crowd in the dream signifies a secret. The two men were readily identified as the dreamer himself and a young man with whom he spent the evening of the night of the dream. The dreamer was treated for homosexuality—passive pederasty—and the murderer of the dream is a young man with whom he is secretly in love. Those of my readers who may be acquainted with dream analysis know that the dagger is a symbol for the penis. Women suffering from lack of sexual gratification often dream of being attacked with knives, daggers, etc. Here the dream shows the realization of a wish to act as a passive pederast for the young man he loves. The stabbing taking place in the heart shows the familiar mechanism of displacement from below to above. The lower part of the body being tabooed, the action is transferred to the upper part; but the mistake very nicely pointed to the patient's true wish; the dagger was plunged into the back.

Other examples showing how dreams solve the problems of the neuroses are the following:

An unmarried woman, Z., of thirty years, was treated by me for hysteria. One of the distressing symptoms was morning nausea with occasional vomiting from which she was suffering from periods of two and three months for the last five years. She stated that she was treated for it during all these years, but without success. I soon concluded that the symptom was hysterical and paid no particular attention to it as it was only one out of many others. One day she told me the following dream:

1. "*I dreamed that Mgt. and I were pregnant and in some way or other I thought that birds were connected with this pregnancy.*

2. "*Then I dreamed of looking down on my own or some one's else bare toes. Each toe became the head of a man as I looked and they all seemed to be smiling or laughing. One of the heads looked like S. V., a male acquaintance.*"

A few facts before proceeding with the analysis. Z. was bi-sexual and since the age of sixteen years had many homosexual amours. Mgt. was her friend with whom she had been in love for years. Mgt. was aware of it and as she is not homosexual they were forced to remain apart. They saw each other now and then and were very friendly. Z. came to me in 1910 and at that time she suffered from fits of depression following periodic debauches of masturbation. Mgt. was the object of her masturbatic fancies.

When I asked her to focus her attention on the idea of pregnancy and repeat her associations she stated that there was a time when she was in mortal dread of being pregnant. At the age of nine years she was seduced by a farm hand and had sexual relations with him. When she was ten years old she heard that girls became pregnant as a result of such relations and she was terrified at the thought of it because she imagined that she was pregnant and that her parents would discover her relations with this man. Her first sexual instructions were received at a very early age. An older child called her attention to the sexual acts of the poultry which she watched with great interest. She imagined that women laid eggs like chickens. The day of the dream she yearned for a child. She spoke with Mgt. about the voidness in their lives and both agreed that they would be contented if they each had a child. She herself had had this wish for years as she is very fond of children. Birds to her mean chickens. She was brought up on a farm and the poultry was always referred to as birds. The first part of the dream, therefore, realized the wish that she and Mgt. were pregnant and the second part of the dream, as will be seen, shows who was responsible for it. When asked to associate to the word "toes" she thought of a foot as this brought to her mind that when she carried on her affair with the farm hand he was in the habit of touching her with his bare feet in forbidden places while the family was sitting around the table. The toe is also a symbol for the penis. The toes resolved themselves into the heads of laughing men and one looked like S. V. because he has a "dirty mind." He has the reputation of being a libertine. He is therefore the right man in the right place and though she consciously rejects him he is accepted by her unconsciously. There are many more subtler determinants for this dream which I am forced to omit here.

At the age of twenty-four she discovered for the first time that pregnancy was accompanied by morning nausea and vomiting. Some time after she began to suffer from the nausea and vomiting. The symptom was therefore the expression of a wish realization and I could definitely show that it came on when the wish was especially strong. With the analysis the symptoms disappeared.

A young married Englishman suffering from a compulsion neurosis was obsessed by the thought of socialism. The obsession came on during the notorious McNamara trial and persisted with increasing vigor until he came to see me a few months ago. No matter in what surrounding he was, whether at his desk or in the theater, he would have to discuss with himself socialism. He would wake up mornings with the question "Is socialism a correct theory, is socialism a true theory of economics?" and he would then argue for and against it. He would read books and pamphlets on the subject, but could never come to any decision. While talking with friends the idea would obtrude itself: "It will be terrible when the government will control everything and some new conditions will come into being which will influence me materially. I wonder whether the president is convinced of the truth of the socialistic doctrines, etc." While attending a play he would be bothered by the idea that it was wrong for him to spend money on luxuries when there were other persons starving. Indeed the patient stated that there was not half an hour when he was free from thoughts on socialism. With the characteristic arguments of *folie raisonant* he went through the most absurd and abstruse argumentations. Lest there should be some misunderstanding I will state that ordinarily the patient had no interest at all in socialism; he professed Catholicism and was quite conservative in his ideas. He realized the absurdity of his compulsive thinking, but was powerless to control it.

After coming to me for a few weeks he brought the following dream: *"Bernard Shaw, the writer, was the guest at some affair and I was there, too. There was another man there who, when he removed his peculiar wig, I noticed was the humorous writer O."*

The determinants of the dream were as follows: A few days before he had read that the Governor General of Jamaica is a socialist and that he once shocked the English aristocracy by inviting Bernard Shaw to one of his social gatherings. The day before the dream he had read a reference to Brieux's play "Damaged Goods," a play dealing with sex to which Bernard Shaw wrote a preface. On continuing the association he recalled the story of "Man and Superman," Shaw's play; how everyone was shocked because a girl was supposed to have been pregnant and how the hero, Tanner, defended her saying that she was going to perform the noblest function of womanhood. He, too, is liberal on the question of sex. The lady's name was Violet. His wife's name is Viola.

According to the rules of association there must have been a close relationship between the sexual lives of Shaw's heroine and his wife and further investigation actually showed that this was so. In brief he admitted that for some time before marriage they led a sexual life and that on a few occasions she had reason to fear pregnancy.

The subject of pregnancy came up again the night before the dream because he imagined that his wife was getting stout. He stated that he did not have the slightest apprehension about it as the proper precautions were taken; that everything was well when he left home a few weeks ago (he returned the day before the dream). He refused to proceed with the associations, but upon being urged he reproduced a rather intimate scene between himself and his wife. For some reason he was depressed and kept on asking his wife "Aren't you all mine, aren't you all mine?" and despite all her assurance he asked the question over and over again. I told him that judging from this scene one would think that he was not sure of his wife's fidelity. He readily admitted that while it did not enter his mind during this scene he has entertained ideas of jealousy since he first became acquainted with his wife. To my question he answered that he is not jealous of any particular man, that the idea is vague and that he suppresses it as soon as it crosses his mind. He then recalled that before he met his wife he was interested in another girl to whom his parents objected. His mother said that "she was a rag on every bush," meaning that she was owned by a great many men. This recalled to him that while he was separated from his wife he met a great many women who were "a rag on every bush." He did not yield to temptation, but entertained a great many forbidden fancies.

The associations making up the elements of the dream thus far reproduced brought to light a complex of marked feeling tone, the content of which is jealousy. He suspected his wife of infidelity, but he has no particular person in mind. It is simply a general jealousy.

When asked about Mr. O. in the dream he stated that he did not know it was Mr. O. until he removed his wig. He is not acquainted personally with O., but knows him by sight. He heard that although O. is married he does not disdain light flirtations when he is away from his wife. He excuses O.'s actions by saying that he belongs to a rather passionate type of man. His description of O. corresponds to himself and when I called his attention to it he at once corroborated it by saying that he was aware of the remarkable resemblance between them and that strangers have noticed it. When I asked him about the wig he stated that O. recently wrote a pseudoscientific paper on hair culture. For many delicate reasons which cannot be explained he himself had of late something to do with hair.

These associations, as well as others that need not be mentioned, not only explain the dream fragment but also the obsession. The dream deals with the most intimate factors of the dreamer's life. In brief he is not sure of his wife, and although he is an admirer of Shaw he is not quite willing to accept his views on sex. He does not believe in freedom of sex, he wants his wife to have no other man beside himself. While he was separated from her he was restrained in his temptation by the thought that he had no right to practise what he would abhor in his wife. He does not believe in collective ownership when it concerns his own wife. In the dream, however, he identifies himself with O., who, according to his belief, is quite free in his marital vows. In other words, what's right for the goose is not necessarily so for the gander. This conflict which existed since his betrothal and which is very painful to him therefore appears under the obsession of socialism which, to our patient, is "collective ownership, common possession." The truth of this assumption was confirmed by the fact that the obsession disappeared as soon as its true meaning became known to the patient.

It is not only in diagnosing gross neurotic symptoms that the dream is of service, but it also helps us to diagnose and cure so-called peculiar traits of character. To illustrate this I will cite the following case:

A young married woman of twenty-six years consulted me and decided to come to me for regular psychanalytic treatment. When she was about to leave she wished to pay me for the consultation. I told her that it was my custom to send monthly statements to my patients and that she might wait until the end of the month before paying me. She thanked me for my offer, but emphatically declared that she would pay at the end of each consultation, adding that she always pays cash, be it to the doctor, druggist, grocer, milliner or dressmaker. Knowing that she was a woman of means I naturally thought it strange and I remarked something to that effect. She then told me that all her friends and acquaintances, including her husband, think that she is peculiar in this respect, but that does not alter her desire not to "run up any bills" and to pay cash for everything. She came to me daily except Sunday and always paid before leaving. After coming to me for a week or two she once forgot to pay, but within a few minutes she returned excitedly and although I was busy with the next patient she insisted upon seeing me. She was very profuse in her apologies despite my assuring her that there was no need for her returning, let alone for apologizing. The following week the same thing happened again with the same results. A week later she actually forgot to pay and did not recall it until she returned home. She telephoned, however, and insisted upon sending my fee to me by special delivery.

Considering the financial experiences we physicians sometimes have with patients I should have had no cause for complaint and that was exactly what one of my colleagues who is interested in psychanalysis thought. But when I asked him the meaning of the patient's extreme scrupulosity he stated that judging by the fact that she had forgotten to pay on a number of occasions it would seem that she was not quite pleased with the treatment and hence did not like to pay for it. His reasoning was in accordance with psychanalytic experience as we are taught that there is no accidental forgetting and that there is always a purpose in forgetting. We usually forget what we do not wish to remember. But I pointed out to him that both she herself and her friends assert that this feeling—"the terrible honesty," as one friend called it—has existed since girlhood so that it could not have any special bearing on her feeling toward the treatment. Moreover, I was very sure that she was satisfied with the progress she was making in the treatment. A few weeks later she brought the following dream: "*I was invited to tea at the house of J., but I did not go. Instead I went with a large party of school girls on some sort of picnic. When it came to be 7 o'clock I was sorry that J. had been waiting for me all the afternoon and knew that I ought to telephone her. I went out to telephone and found that I had no money. I saw a gold piece lying before me. I knew to whom it belonged, in fact people were looking for it, but as I needed money to telephone I did not give it up. I knew I was a thief and I was sorry, but I kept the money just the same. Then I began to borrow everything—money, gloves, etc.—and people all seemed to be afraid I would not return the things I borrowed.*"

For many reasons I am only giving a fragment of a long dream, but it will suffice to demonstrate what I wish to point out. The dream was determined by the following experiences of the day before: She was invited to a tea and did not like to go. She received a letter from a schoolmate inviting her to visit her. She had some conversation about money matters with her husband. There were many associations which I shall omit as not absolutely necessary and will confine myself to those directly bearing on the complex. When I asked her to focus her attention on the gold piece she suddenly became very emotional. She begged me not to press her to tell me this particular thought as it was very painful, etc., etc. After much argument and protest she gave the following associations: Her mother was not faithful to her father, and as he was frequently away on business she entertained many intrigues. It was when my patient was a little girl of about seven or eight years that she came into the room unobserved by her mother and saw the latter going through the pockets of one of her paramours who was too intoxicated to protest. She left as she entered, but she never forgave her mother for it. She said nothing, but for a long time she felt a strong resentment and aversion toward her mother. Nevertheless, shortly after while at school she imitated her mother by stealing a few pennies from a classmate's pocket. She was never discovered and she never stole anything else and soon thereafter, at the age of ten or eleven years, became a model of honesty.

This dream may be called a reaction dream as it shows the reverse side of the person and explains that our dreamer's "terrible honesty" is simply a reaction to her unconscious dishonesty. This patient identified herself with her mother in almost every respect. She led the same life as her mother and treated her husband just as her mother treated her father. The picture would have been the same had she continued to show a tendency to dishonesty, but as this was repressed, the reaction had to be a scrupulous honesty. Like the character in Ibsen's "Pillars of Society" she had "to hold up the banner of the ideal." That accounts for the fact that she often forgot to pay, as she actually desired. For some time before the analysis of this dream she would pay in advance to make sure that she would not forget. The conversation with her husband was about her allowance. She asked for more and he granted her request. Owing to the fact that she was at the time in love with another man her conscience pricked her and she said to herself: "I am nothing but a thief and I have no right to his money." This was the main determinant of the dream. After everything was analyzed and her unconscious complex was laid bare to her she was quite willing to "run up" a bill with me.

Having referred so often to symbols in dreams it will not be amiss to say a few words about symbolism in general. Madeline Pelletier defines a symbol as "a false perception of a marked relation of identity or analogy between two objects which, in reality, present only a vague analogy." This definition is confirmed by the study of philology. Primitive writing consisted of a collection of symbols; the Egyptians, for example, used figures to represent ideas and the original alphabet consisted of a collection of symbols. Thus the original letter B did not stand for the consonant, but it was a picture of a crude outline of a house and meant to represent the idea "house." With the advance of civilization the alphabetic symbols lost their original meaning and became consonants and vowels. Symbols, therefore, represent a lower form of thinking for they identify objects which have only a very remote. analogy. Children and primitive races still make use of this form of expression. Thus a child calls a stick a horse simply because it can ride on it. The analogy between the stick and the horse is very remote indeed. As the child grows older and becomes able to discriminate and compare it no longer forms such vague analogies. The symbols that we use in our daily life though more complex and specialized are symbols none the less. The Statue of Liberty, the cross, the masonic emblems, the barber's pole, are examples of this nature. Language is full of symbols. A symbol is a form of short-hand writing. One word may express an idea or have many meanings, *e.g.*, the word "green" may represent a color or stand for the idea hope. Religion swarms with symbolisms and the more primitive the form the more prolific the symbolism. It has also been found that diminished attention favors a lower form of thinking and that a disturbance of attention causes shallow reaction types. This accounts for symbolization in hallucinations, delusions, dreams, wit and poetry;* that is, one is apt to find symbols in all those productions that come from unconscious activities. When we have our full attention and can compare and discriminate we are not likely to form any remote analogies. On the other hand, whenever these factors are disturbed or absent, as in dreams and psychoses, and under certain conditions even in the waking state, we make use of symbols. In this connection the following experience related by an acquaintance will be of interest: While walking with two friends their attention was attracted by a big bird in the distant height. One of them suggested that it was a crow and remarked that it was rather unusual to see this bird in the city. As it came nearer they were sure that it was

* An excellent paper on Poetry and Dreams was published by Professor F. C. Prescott in the Journal of Abnormal Psychology, Vol. VII, 1 and 2.

a stray or escaped eagle, and finally it turned out to be a flying machine. The reason for these mistakes at first was the inability to judge and discriminate, and had they left before the machine came near enough to afford the opportunity for proper comparison and judgment they would have been convinced that they saw a crow or an eagle.

During my service in the Clinic of Psychiatry at Zurich I was often present while my former chief Prof. Bleuler examined the patients. One of the tests, principally for attention, was to expose very rapidly pictures and ask the patient to tell what he saw. The pictures used were from a booklet containing over two hundred pictures, both simple and complex, of everything imaginable. Among the pictures of the vegetables was the asparagus and whenever the latter was rapidly exposed the patients almost always believed that it was the penis. I have repeated this same test hundreds of times with the same result. The patients are shown more than ninety pictures before they get to the picture of the asparagus and whether the answers are correct or not they are usually given promptly. When the asparagus is shown they invariably hesitate; some give no answer at all; their expression, however, plainly betrays their thoughts. Others claim that they have not seen distinctly enough, and some of the bolder ones simply laugh. It is also interesting to watch their features when they discover the real picture. Some are plainly disappointed, others are very relieved, and, lately, one patient exclaimed, "I didn't know I was so evil-minded." They all admitted that they first thought of the penis. Here the mistake is plainly due to an inability to discriminate between two objects having a vague resemblance, and is caused by insufficient attention owing to the rapid exposure. It is such vague analogies which, when found in dreams we call symbols, which have given cause to so much controversy. Those who find it so strange should remember that we are not even pioneers in the use of symbolism, but like in a great many other things we pay attention to something which our opponents never think worth examining. That so many symbolic expressions in dreams are sexual is not at all surprising when we consider the enormous symbolization of sex in the waking state. Let those who object to sexual symbols in dreams reflect for a moment and they will soon find any number of sex symbols in their own conscious minds. Because sex is the strongest impulse we possess it has been subjected to constant suppression and for that reason one finds it symbolized and otherwise in the unconscious and in literature. When the poet says "And Maidens, becoming bottles, cry aloud for corks" (Pope—The Rape of the Lock), he uses gross sexual symbols concerning which there can be no mistake. I have found the very same and similar symbols in many dreams. In the unconscious productions there is no limit to sexual symbolization. Kleinpaul justly remarked "Man sexualizes the universe." An examination of our colloquialisms, stage wit, popular songs, etc., will convince one of the truth of this statement.

To illustrate how the dream makes use of symbolisms I will cite the following dream. A woman of forty years related this dream: "*I saw my son L. jammed in the fireplace and tried to get him out, but I couldn't. I was awfully frightened and called out 'Papa, papa.'*" She laughingly added, "You will probably find something sexual in it."

When the dreamer finds it necessary to add such a

remark it is always well to think of the saying "Many a truth is said in jest." When I questioned her about the dream she stated that "papa" in the dream did not mean her father but her lodger, who is so nicknamed. As she could give no associations to "fireplace" I took it to be a symbol for the vagina. The other facts are as follows: This woman has been a grass widow for years and suffered much from lack of sexual gratification. She was anxious to enter into an amour with "Papa," but was deterred by the fear of pregnancy. She had an affair before and had to go through a rather bad abortion. Her son who was in the fireplace in the dream is nineteen years old. She recalled that when she became pregnant with him she went through a severe hysterical attack. She was afraid of pregnancy and childbirth and implored her family physician to produce an abortion. He refused to help her so she herself tried everything she knew of, but to no avail. The dream, therefore, repeats an incident of nineteen years ago. At that time her son was jammed in the "fireplace" and she couldn't get him out. For the previous few weeks she was occupied with a similar situation. She often said to herself "if he (Papa) would take care, I would have nothing to fear." In the dream she actually calls upon him to do this, but the erstwhile embryo is replaced by her son as he is now.

The symbolism in the dream is the same to-day as it was in the Biblical times when Joseph acted the part of the oneiroscopist, and as we still see it in the dream books. But whereas the ancients and the laity of to-day ignore their own subjective mind and seek interpretation from magicians and dream books we allow the dreamer to interpret his own dreams and to find the symbolisms in his own mind. What we do is simply to call his attention to the different connections which he himself generally cannot see because of his own critique, prejudices and resistances.

We also differ from the ancients and laity by not seeing in the dream the future, but rather the past. Yet, in a way, the dream is also related to the future inasmuch as its fulfilled wish represents what we are striving for. This, in my opinion, explains the ancient and modern superstition regarding the future realization of dreams. It has its origin in incidents resembling the dream of Miss G. and those of the children mentioned before. Thus both children forced their parents to fulfil their wishes. In order to appease her little girl the mother had to procure for her some chocolate almonds and the boy did not stop crying until his mother gave him the money of his dream.

There are dreams which continue to manifest themselves for weeks and months until the wish they contain is actually realized. A chronic alcoholic showing delusions of jealousy disliked a dog because his wife "was more attached to the dog than to him." He continued to dream at different times that the dog was run over, taken away by the dogcatcher, etc., until one day during his wife's absence he really disposed of it. Here the dream ostensibly treated of the future, at least so the wife thought on her return home. "Poor Fido," she exclaimed, "John (husband) dreamed only last week that he was caught by the dogcatchers and now the dream has come true." This is the so-called resolution dream.[13] The person resolves, perhaps unconsciously, to do a certain thing and the dream continues to represent it as realized until it is actually accomplished. This explains the mechanism of the "dreams that come true." I have analyzed a number of such dreams and all showed that the wish always preceded the event in question. Thus one of my patients dreamed that her brother who lived in another city was dead, and after relating her dream to her husband received word that her brother had really died. The analysis showed that her brother suffered from chronic tuberculosis which the doctors declared fatal months before. She was fully aware of the gravity of his malady and often thought that he would be better off dead than alive. Her mother lived with her, but, owing to her brother's illness she stayed with him. She was nearing the end of a pregnancy and daily hoped that her mother would return before her confinement. This recalled similar experiences of childhood when her mother often neglected her for the same brother because he was very delicate and sickly. As a child she often wished him dead, a thing quite common among children to whom the idea of death means simply to be away. The conscious wish "he would be better off dead than alive" became the dream incitor because it succeeded in arousing a similar infantile wish. For, as Freud says, "The conscious wish becomes a dream incitor only when it succeeds in arousing a similar unconscious one," and "The wish as represented in the dream must be an infantile one."[14]

The realization of our waking dreams shows precisely the same mechanisms. This can be observed not only in the individual, but in whole races. We all know that the

Leitmotif of orthodox Judaism is and always has been the reestablishment of a Jewish nationality, the "return to Jerusalem"; and should Zionism ever succeed in obtaining Palestine, the Biblical dreams, the prophecies would be considered as having "come true." Popular language expresses the idea in the saying "Where there is a will there is a way."

These brief analyses distinctly show the connection between the dream and the neuroses. I am quite convinced that had we not analyzed the dream, the psychic conflicts underlying the neurosis of Miss G. could not have been discovered, as they were unconscious to the patient, and that she would have merged into a chronic neurosis. Very soon after the complexes were discovered and brought to her consciousness her symptoms began to disappear and within two months she was perfectly cured. It must be added that besides analyzing the dream her other symptoms had to be explained to her. Thus her abnormal attachment to her mother disappeared as soon as she became conscious of the fact that it was hiding a repressed wish that her mother might die so that she could use the estate to assist Mr. F. The insight and psychological education which she gained during the analysis also helped her to overcome some of her false pride and prudishness, and as a result she is now happily married to Mr. F. Thus her wish was realized.

RÉSUME

1. As Freud has shown, dreams are perfect psychological mechanisms. They have a definite meaning and contain a wish fulfilment.

2. Every psychotic symptom is the expression of a former mental occurrence and symbolically represents a wish fulfilment.

3. The repression of the unconscious is at the basis of both the dream and the psychotic symptom.

4. Dreams are the product of the unconscious and hence afford the easiest access to the exploration of the neurosis.

References

1. Sante de Sanctis. Les Maladies mental et les rêves, 1897. Extrait des Annales de la Société de médecine de Gand.

Ideler: Ueber die Entstehung des Wahnsinns aus Träumen. Charité Annalen, III, p. 284, 1862.

Féré: A Contribution to the Pathology of Dreams. Brain, IX, 1887.

Lasègue: Le Delire alcoolique n'est pas un delire mais un rêve. Archives général de médecine, 1881.

Sully, J.: The Dream as a Revelation. Fortnightly Review, March, 1893.

2. Freud: The Interpretation of Dreams. George Allan Co., London, and The Macmillan Co., New York. Translated by A. A. Brill.

3. Freud: Selected Papers on Hysteria and Psychoneurosis. Translated by A. A. Brill, Monograph Series of Journal of Nervous and Mental Dis. Co.

4. Jung: The Psychology of Dementia Præcox. Translated by Peterson and Brill, Monograph Series Journal of Nervous and Mental Dis. Co.

5. Freud: Die Psychopathologie des Alltagsleben. Karger, Berlin. *Cf.* also Chap. VII.

6. *Cf.* Chap. V.

7. For the mechanism of jokes *cf.* Chap. XII.

8. *Cf.* Chap. III.

9. For an excellent example of this mechanism see Chap. I, p. 29.

10. Stekel, W.: Nervöse Angstzustände und ihre Behandlung, p. 117.

11. Die Diagnose der Homosexualität, Neurolog. Zentralbl., 1908, p. 338.

12. *Cf.* Chap. V.

13. Freud: Sammlung kleiner Schriften zur Neurosenlehre, Zweite Folge, p. 59, Deuticke, Wien, 1909.

14. Freud: The Interpretation of Dreams. Chap. VII.

CHAPTER III

THE ACTUAL NEUROSES

Neurasthenia and Anxiety Neurosis; their Symptoms, Mechanism, Etiology and Relation to the Psychoneuroses

Freud divides the neuroses into psycho and actual neuroses. The psychoneuroses comprise hysteria and compulsion neurosis (doubts, obsessions and phobias) while the actual neuroses include neurasthenia and anxiety neurosis. The sexual life plays an important part in the determination of both classes. But whereas hysteria and compulsion neurosis are altogether of a psychogenetic origin, neurasthenia and anxiety neurosis are due to somatic sexual injuries.

As the typical symptoms of neurasthenia Freud mentions headache, or pressure in the head, spinal irritation, and dyspepsia with flatulence, and constipation. By adhering closely to these symptoms one can easily differentiate the real neurasthenia from the pseudo-neurasthenias such as the organically determined nasal reflex neurosis, the neurotic disturbances of cachexias and arteriosclerosis, the early stages of progressive paralysis, and some of the psychoses. Concerning the etiology Freud says "Neurasthenia always originates whenever the adequate (action) unburdening is replaced by a less adequate one, like the normal coitus under the most favorable conditions by a masturbation or spontaneous pollution."[1]

Bearing in mind this symptom-complex, neurasthenia ceases to be the "big garbage can," as Forel fitly calls it, and becomes a rather limited entity. For it is known to every observer in this field that neurasthenia in the generally accepted sense may comprise almost anything from anxiety neurosis to psychoses proper. Well developed cases of dementia præcox, paresis and other psychoses are often diagnosed and treated for months, even years, as neurasthenics.

That anxiety plays a part in the neuroses was fully recognized by almost all writers on this subject; but its isolation into a separate entity and its reference to a special sexual etiology was first established by Freud in his dissertation, "On the Right to Separate from Neurasthenia a Definite Symptom Complex as Anxiety Neurosis."[2]

Before going into the etiology of anxiety neurosis I will first enumerate the clinical symptoms which are as follows:

1. General irritability. This frequent symptom especially expresses itself in auditory hyperesthesia and is a frequent cause of insomnia of which more than one form belongs to anxiety neurosis.

2. Anxious expectation which manifests itself in an uneasiness and a tendency to pessimistic conception of things, or in a tendency to "make mountains out of mole hills." Persons showing this symptom evince a frequent tendency to pangs of conscience, scrupulosity and pedantry. Thus a man who suffered from anxious expectation thought that something might have happened to his mother because there was a thunder-storm while she

was riding in a train. He was anxiously waiting for news of some disaster and was not relieved until he heard that she had reached her destination. Anxious expectation is the most essential symptom of the neurosis. There seems to be a quantum of freely floating anxiety which is forever ready to unite itself with suitable ideations.

3. Anxiousness can also suddenly break into consciousness without being aroused by the issue of an idea. Such attacks consist either of the anxious feeling alone without any associated idea or of the nearest interpretation of the termination of life, such as ideas of sudden death or threatening insanity, or the anxious feeling may be combined with a disturbance of one or many somatic functions, such as respiration, cardiac activity, the vasomotor innervation and the glandular activity. The patient may complain of "heart spasm," "heavy breathing," "inordinate appetite," "profuse perspiration," "feeling badly," etc.

4. The amount of admixture of these elements varies extraordinarily and any accompanying symptom may alone constitute the attack. Accordingly there are rudimentary attacks of anxiety and equivalents for the attack of anxiety. The following equivalents may be mentioned:

(*a*) Attacks of disturbance of heart action, ranging from palpitation, transitory arhythmia, with longer continued tachycardia to grave states of heart weakness. These are not always easy to differentiate from organic heart affections. It may manifest itself in pseudo-angina pectoris, a delicate diagnostic sphere.

(*b*) Attacks of respiratory disturbances, many forms of nervous dyspnœa and asthma-like attacks.

(*c*) Attacks of profuse perspiration, often nocturnal.

(*d*) Attacks of trembling and shaking which may be readily mistaken for hysterical attacks.

(*e*) Attacks of inordinate appetite, often combined with dizziness.

(*f*) Attacks of diarrhœa.

(*g*) Attacks of locomotor dizziness.

(*h*) Attacks of congestion embracing also the so-called vasomotor neurasthenia.

(*i*) Attacks of paresthesias (these are seldom without anxiety or a similar discomfort).

(*j*) Sudden terrified awakening.

(*k*) Frequency of micturition.

(*l*) Cramplike muscular attacks.

5. Nocturnal frights (pavor nocturnus of adults) usually accompanied by anxiety, dyspnœa, perspiration, etc., are only a variety of the anxiety attack and determine a second form of insomnia in the sphere of anxiety neurosis. The pavor nocturnus of children belongs to the same neurosis.

6. A prominent symptom of anxiety neurosis is vertigo which in its lightest form may be designated as "dizziness." Attacks of vertigo with or without fear belong to the gravest symptoms of the neurosis. This form of vertigo is neither a rotatory dizziness nor is it confined to certain planes or lines like Menier's vertigo. It consists in a specific feeling of discomfort accompanied by sensations of a heaving ground, sinking legs, of the impossibility of remaining in an upright position, and at the same time there is a feeling that the legs are as heavy as lead, that they shake and give way. This vertigo never leads to falling.

7. Two groups of typical phobias develop on the basis of the chronic anxiousness (anxious expectation) on the one hand, and the tendency to vertiginous anxiety attacks on the other. In the first group we have the fear for snakes, thunderstorms, darkness, vermin, etc., as well as the typical moral overscrupulousness and the forms of *folie du doute*. The available fear is here used to strengthen the instinctive aversions implanted in every man. The second group comprises agoraphobia with all its accessory forms, all of which are characterized by their relation to locomotion. The phobia is usually. determined by a precedent attack of vertigo.

8. The disturbances of the digestive functions are few, but are characteristic. One often finds the sensations of nausea and sickly feeling. The symptom of inordinate appetite with or without congestion may serve as a rudimentary attack of anxiety. The tendency to diarrhœa which is a chronic alteration analogous to the anxious expectation has occasioned the queerest diagnostic mistakes.

9. The paresthesias which accompany the attacks of vertigo or anxiety associate themselves into a firm sequence resembling the sensation of the hysterical aura. These associated sensations are changeable and atypical, but they sometimes become converted into physical sensations like rheumatic pains.

THE OCCURRENCE AND ETIOLOGY OF ANXIETY NEUROSIS

In some cases of anxiety neurosis no etiology can be readily found, but in such cases one can usually find a marked hereditary taint. Whenever the neurosis is acquired one can always find "that the etiologically effective factors are based on a series of injuries and influences from the sexual life."[3] These injuries and influences may be either found alone or are reinforced by other banal injuries.

To give a more precise description of the etiological determinants of anxiety neurosis Freud separates those occurring in men from those occurring in women. Regardless of disposition anxiety neurosis appears in women under the following forms:

(*a*) As virginal fear or anxiety in adults. Many definite observations show that an anxiety neurosis almost typically combined with hysteria can be evoked in maturing girls at their first encounter with the sexual problem, either through seeing or through hearing or reading of sex.

(*b*) As fear in the newly married. Young women who remain anesthetic during the first coitus often merge into an anxiety neurosis which disappears after the anesthesia is replaced by normal feeling.

(*c*) As fear in women whose husbands suffer from ejaculatio precox or from diminished potency; and

(*d*) In those whose husbands practice coitus interruptus or reservatus. These cases go together for they only depend on whether the woman attains gratification during coitus or not. The determinant for the origin of the anxiety neurosis is found in the latter case. But if the husband suffering from ejaculatio præcox can repeat coitus with better results immediately thereafter the wife will not merge into the neurosis. Coitus interruptus is only injurious for the wife if the husband interrupts coitus as soon as he is about to ejaculate without concerning himself about bringing to an end the excitement of his wife. If he waits until his wife is gratified the process has the same effect on her as normal coitus, but then he becomes afflicted with anxiety neurosis. I have on record more than eighty cases which fully confirm the above statements.

(*e*) As anxiety in widows and intentional abstainers, often in typical combination with obsessions, and

(*f*) As anxiety in the climacterium during the last marked enhancement of the sexual impulse.

The forms (*c*), (*d*) and (*e*) contain the determinants under which the anxiety neurosis originates in the female most frequently and most independently of hereditary predisposition. The determinants of anxiety neurosis in the male find their analogy in the female and are formulated into the following groups:

(*a*) Anxiety of the intentional abstainer; this is frequently combined with symptoms of defense (obsessions, hysteria).

(*b*) Anxiety in men with frustrated excitement (during the engagement period); persons who fearing the consequences of sexual relations gratify themselves by handling and looking at the woman. These determinants hold true also for the woman (prolonged engagements with frustrated excitement) and furnish the purest cases of anxiety neurosis.

(*c*) Anxiety in men who practise coitus interruptus. This form of coitus injures the woman if practised regardless of her gratification, but it may also injure the man if in order to gratify his wife he voluntarily controls coitus by delaying the ejaculation.

(*d*) Anxiety in men during the period of senility. Some

men go through a climacterium like women and may merge into an anxiety neurosis when their potency diminishes and their libido increases. This case and (*c*) hold true for both sexes.

(*e*) Masturbating neurasthenics merge into anxiety neurosis as soon as they stop masturbating as their former life has made them especially unfit to lead a life of abstinence.

(*f*) This last determinant is really not of a sexual nature. Both sexes may merge into anxiety neurosis through considerable overwork, exhaustive exertion such as sleepless nights, nursing the sick or even serious illnesses.

The facts thus far enumerated go to show that in anxiety neurosis we deal with an accumulation of sexual excitement and that the anxiety underlying the manifestations of the neurosis is not of psychic, but of somatic origin. Moreover, since it has been found that a whole series of cases of this neurosis shows marked diminution of the sexual desire, to an extent, that on revealing to the patients that their affliction depends on "insufficient gratification" they regularly reply that this is impossible as just now their whole desire is extinguished—all these indications favor the assumption "that the mechanism of the anxiety neurosis is to be found in the deviation of the somatic sexual excitement from the psychic and in the abnormal utilization of this excitement caused thereby."[4]

Hence we see that the actual neuroses, neurasthenia and anxiety neurosis, differ materially from the psychoneuroses, compulsion neurosis and hysteria. The latter group are due to purely psychogenetic factors, while the first are due to somatic sexual injuries.

I have pointed out above that the characteristic factor of hysteria, according to Freud, is the ability to convert the psychic into the physical. That is, whenever we find the classical symptoms of hysteria, such as paralyses, contractures, aphonias, convulsions, astasia abasia, etc., we deal with a conversion hysteria. In contradistinction to this, the symptoms due to somatic sexual injuries belong to anxiety neurosis.

It was found, however, that no definite lines could be drawn; that besides the somatic sexual injuries the anxiety neuroses also showed a psychic mechanism. This psychic mechanism is the same as in hysteria, but instead of conversion into physical symptoms there is anxiety. "The anxiety is, as it were, the only symptom into which the psychic excitement is converted." The etiology, the rôle of repression and the psychic processes are the same as in hysteria. For this new class of cases Freud suggested the term "anxiety hysteria" and the whole group was first described by Stekel in his interesting and instructive book.[5]

My own experience, based on the observation of a great many cases of anxiety neurosis taught me that there is a psychic element in almost all cases. I could demonstrate it in nearly all my cases and I must confess that, owing to lack of opportunity and personal resistances (it concerned elderly illiterate patients from clinical dispensary practice) I did not try hard enough to ascertain the true circumstances in the others. I can say, however, that even those patients were cured and some greatly benefited by advising them properly concerning their sexual lives.

I do not hesitate to advise the use of the condom when it is a question of coitus interruptus. The condom properly used—lubrication of penis and moistening or lubrication of condom after it is in place—is the nearest substitute for normal coitus.

It would lead me too far afield to enter here into a deep discussion on the subject of masturbation. I will simply state that years of study and personal investigation have taught me that as masturbation is practically universal it cannot be considered the terrible demon it is painted to be by some. I fully agree with those who claim that masturbation does not in any way injure the brain or cord. I have seen many cases who were supposed to have been harmed by masturbation, but careful investigation showed beyond any doubt that masturbation had no direct bearing on the condition in question. Whatever harm masturbation may do is mostly produced indirectly by the constant struggle which accompanies it. The patients are terrified by reading quack literature and, I regret to say, by some uninformed doctors. They are threatened with "paralysis," "paresis," "consumption of the spine," etc., and as a result they become depressed, hypochondriacal and self-conscious. But as soon as they are convinced that they are not doomed and that masturbation cannot cause any insanity or the other dreadful maladies they soon lose most of their symptoms. Nor must it be imagined that robbing masturbation of its horrors encourages its practice. On the contrary, I found that as long as the patients dread it and struggle against it they masturbate twice as often as when they become convinced that it has none of its former supposed horrors. For it makes no difference whether we occupy ourselves with sex in a positive or negative way the result is the same. It is stimulated to greater activity. Moreover, many patients masturbate very often because they are sure that masturbation caused an enfeeblement of their will power and hence there is no use resisting. As they become enlightened the practice gradually decreases, and as the patient has no need for constantly occupying himself with sexual ideas there is less tension to be removed.

There is a class of masturbators, however, who may be designated as chronic because they continue the practice throughout their whole life. They usually belong to the psychopathic type and the masturbation must be considered a result rather than a cause of the condition.

As I said before in almost all these cases there is a psychic element and when this is found we must not only correct the abnormal sexual life, but to cure the patient we must resort, in addition, to psychanalysis. As an example of an anxiety hysteria of this type I will give the following case:

Mrs. L., thirty-eight years old, Austrian, married, having four healthy children, was seen by me in the department of psychiatry in the Vanderbilt Clinic in October, 1908. She complained of nervousness, depression, anxiety and insomnia from which she suffered for about two weeks. On questioning her I found that this was her sixth attack, that the first attack came on six years ago and repeated itself annually, usually lasting about two months. Like the doctor who saw her before me I thought of manic depressive insanity, but on closer examination I changed my diagnosis to anxiety hysteria. Her family history was negative. She herself claimed that she was never sick before her present illness. Anthropologically and otherwise she corresponded to her type—Austrian Jewess. Physically there was nothing worthy of note.

When I asked her to tell me her chief complaint she said that it was a depression and anxiety. She stated that her attacks were not all alike. Thus, her first attack began very suddenly and was characterized by marked anxiety, depression, apprehension and insomnia. The second, third and fourth attacks were considerably milder, the depression being the main symptom, while her fifth attack again showed the anxiety and insomnia. Her symptoms did not in any way incapacitate her. She attended to her housework as usual and there was absolutely no psychomotor retardation. She maintained, however, that she was afraid that something would happen to her and that she often cried out without knowing why. There were no distinct phobias, but in all her attacks she showed the characteristic *folie du doute.* Thus, during her attacks she often got out of bed "at least a dozen times" to ascertain whether the door was properly locked or whether the gas was turned off. Besides the symptoms enumerated she also showed the aforecited cardinal symptoms of anxiety neurosis. What influenced me in diagnosticating anxiety hysteria was the typical sexual etiology. The first attack came two years after her husband left for the United States, during which time she lived a virtuous life. For the following three years, while with her husband, she gave birth to two children and thus her emotional needs were fully satisfied. After the fourth child was born she wanted no more children and her husband practised coitus interruptus. That seemed to account for the difference in the symptoms of the various attacks. For lack of gratification is a very frequent cause of insomnia, particularly in persons showing nothing else to account for it. But, of course, we have not accounted for the depression which was present in every attack.

As soon as I decided on the diagnosis I proceeded with the psychanalysis. I usually begin by asking the patient to give me a full account of the origin of the disease. She knew that the first attack came on about six years before, just before she came to the United States. Her husband left her in Austria with two children and after having been away for about two years he sent for her to join him in New York. It was while she was getting ready for her journey that the first attack came on and continued for about two months. She was quite certain that it had no connection with her leaving Austria; on the contrary she was more than glad to join her husband. The subsequent attacks came on periodically every fall. She also recalled that her attacks came together with the Jewish fall holidays. More than this she did not know. I attempted an association experiment, but either she refused her cooperation or she was unable to grasp the meaning of the procedure. As I attributed her depression and anxiety to the repression of painful or disagreeable reminiscences, and as the dream is the *via regia* to the unconscious or the repression I asked her to tell me something of her dreams. She insisted that she had not dreamed for years. She finally recalled, however, having had a dream before or at the beginning of her first attack. This was the dream:

"*I walked on the street and a horse harnessed to a wagon was running toward me. I could not get out of its way; the horse was almost upon me. I put out my arm to push it away when it caught my hand in its mouth and bit me. Screaming, I awoke terrified.*"

These were the "manifest thoughts" of the dream and to those acquainted with Freud's theories they are quite significant. In analyzing dreams we simply translate the manifest into the latent. The manifest thoughts have apparently no meaning, but the latent thoughts are senseful and always show the hidden fulfilment of a repressed wish. As the dream occurred before or at the onset of the attack I assumed that it had some relation to it, as dreams are always based on experiences or thoughts of the day preceding the dream. Also, the fear in the dream pointed to its being of a sexual nature and I suspected that the horse was simply a sexual symbol.[6]

On asking the patient to tell something about the horse she stated that it was a bay horse and very spirited. That was all she knew. When I urged her to tell me all the thoughts that occurred to her in this connection she impatiently remarked: "I don't know what to tell you; I could talk about horses for hours. I know quite a bit about horses, as I lived next door to a government horse-breeding station." She then displayed considerable emotivity, but on being urged to tell whatever was in her mind she stated that she witnessed the practical details of horse breeding at a very early age. Indeed, she was certain that this was her first conscious sexual impression. "Of course," she added, "I was too young to know the real meaning of things. I imagined that the horses were fighting." This sadistic conception is very common in children and as Freud shows in his paper, "Concerning Infantile Sexual Theories,"[7] children always interpret the sexual act in that sense. There was a sudden blocking and when asked to continue she suddenly recalled something which had no connection with horses. The evening before the dream, while sitting in the room with some neighbors, some animal, perhaps a mouse or rat, ran out of the brick stove into the bed. Unlike her sex she was ordinarily not afraid of mice or rats, but this time she was terribly frightened and continued to be so for hours. She rummaged through the bed and found nothing; still she was afraid to sleep in this bed. This recalled that this attack of fright occurred a few hours after an unsuccessful attempt to sell her feather beds. She again became silent and claimed that her stream of thoughts was exhausted. Suspecting that her attack of fear was the manifestation of a mental conflict in a sexual abstainer, I asked her why she was so terrified at the sight of what she imagined was a mouse or rat, if she was ordinarily not afraid of these animals. Her ready response was that she was never afraid of the real mouse or rat, but that at that time she imagined that they were only apparitions, that someone tried to exert some evil influence over her by magic. She laughingly added that she no longer believed in such nonsense. When I asked her who she thought tried to exert an evil influence over her and why that was attempted, she at first refused to answer, remarking that the whole thing was not worth talking about, but after considerable urging she said that she then believed that it was a man who offered to buy her feather beds. With great emotivity and hesitation she described this man, whom we will call X. as a very disagreeable and impudent fellow. He wished to buy her feather beds, but for some reason she could not come to any terms with him. He, however, persisted in calling on her until she became so tired of seeing him that she hid herself whenever she saw him coming. She suddenly broke off the narrative and when I urged her to continue she became very indignant. She said she saw no reason for the revival of all this foolishness; she was very sure that this questioning had nothing to do with her disease, etc., etc. Such outbursts are very frequent in the course of psychanalysis and always occur when we strike the main complex.[8]

As soon as I knew the circumstances of the case, and after hearing the dream, I thought of *cherchez l'homme*, and after witnessing her emotional outburst I was sure that I had my man. As I said above the dream showed a mental conflict of a sexual nature and the attack of fear, too, as I will show later, symbolically represented a sexual attack. Indeed the whole setting was such that there was no doubt in my mind that she had some sexual experience with X., and that her periodic attacks of depression merely represented the former libido changed into depression by repression.

After calming her I frankly told her that I was convinced that she was concealing something, that I believed she had had some affair with X. and that unless she told me everything I could do nothing for her. She emphatically denied my assumptions, but would not explain why she had to hide when she saw X. and why she thought he tried to exert evil influences over her. She became very indignant when I was equally assertive in my statements and left me rather abruptly. I made no attempt to restrain her or remonstrate with her because my experience taught me that it is of no avail, and that it is well to give the patient a chance to fully discharge her repressed emotions.

Two days later she returned, but this time she looked quite dejected and penitent. A few kind remarks from me helped her to disburden herself. Weeping, she made the following confession: "Since I left you I was very miserable. I have cried most of the time; the whole thing came back to me, I could not banish it from my mind, so I decided to come and tell you all." She then assured me that for the two years that she was separated from her husband she had lived a virtuous life. She was hardly ever bothered by erotic thoughts and had no difficulty in suppressing them when they came. While getting ready to join her husband in America she sold her household effects and X. wanted to buy her feather beds. When she showed him the feather beds he joked with her about her coming journey to America and alluded to her future happiness with her husband. This aroused some erotic thoughts and when X. accompanied his talk by touching her suggestively she was surprised not to have resented it. In brief, she met him a number of times, always on the pretense of selling the feather beds and she was afterward surprised at her own weakness. She, however, assured me that she had not broken her marriage vows. "That is the only thing I have not done," she said. It was after she suddenly awoke to the gravity of the situation that she refused to see him and feared him. She was really afraid of herself; she did not trust herself. These experiences which gave rise to a number of erotic thoughts and fancies were then changed into displeasure. It was then that she was afraid to sleep alone with her children and had to ask a neighbor to sleep with her. It was about the same time that the rat incident occurred which made her think of magic. This was due to the fact that even after she stopped seeing X. she continued to have sexual thoughts and fancies. The more she tried to banish them the more they came. By association of ideas they recalled to her all her sexual experiences, such as early masturbation, etc., which in view of their persistence against her own will she could attribute only to some external power—magic. Of course, it must be remembered that there was a time in her life when she actually believed in magical influence, and owing to the mental upset the repressed complex simply came to the surface. Similar mechanisms are at the basis of hallucinations and delusions.[9]

The other mechanisms of the case are quite simple. As I said above the nature of the dream shows that it deals with sexual emotions. We also showed that the horse was intimately connected with her first sexual impressions. She also stated that when she masturbated later in life the horse often served to arouse her sexual fancies. In the dream when "the horse was almost upon her," *i.e.*, when she almost yielded to temptation, her moral self gained the upper hand and she "put out her arm to push it away." She, however, sustained a scar, her hand was bitten. That part of the dream is constellated by the following facts: She was actually bitten by a horse at the age of six; and her early observations of horse breeding had often excited her passions and induced a repetition of her habits. The same effect had been produced in her by the visits of X. The horse in the dream may therefore be taken in this sense as symbolizing X. who recalls her early impressions of sexuality. The dream often makes use of such symbolizations. The gross sexual is always under repression, hence we see instead its inrooted associations. Horses, bulls, dogs, cats and chickens are often sexual symbols in dreams, because it is with these animals that children are first apt to see the sexual procedures.[10] Our patient conceived sexual relations in the sadistic sense, they were first impressed upon her in childhood by the breeding observations above referred to. In brief, her dream merely symbolizes these relations as shown by the cited association and the expression "the horse was almost upon me." The biting, too, she vividly recalled seeing while watching the horses. The dream, therefore, represents the hidden fulfilment of her repressed wish, while the fear is the libido which was changed by the repression.

It still remains to explain why the depressions continued to recur annually. The incidents enumerated above took place before the Jewish Day of Atonement, and it was on this day, which is the most solemn day for the orthodox Jew, that her actions appeared to her in the most lurid colors. This is the day on which all true believers are inscribed in the "Book of Life" or "Book of Death." It is a day of fasting and confession and she certainly had a lot to confess. She could not consider her sins forgiven, and dreaded some impending evil, perhaps an accident at sea. She came to the United States about five weeks later. She was still in a state of depression, but it soon wore off. But every year, with the approach of this solemn day, the depression returned. She merely celebrated the anniversary of her painful experience. She never recalled the original episode because it was of a disagreeable and painful nature; the accompanying emotions, however, came to the surface and constituted the depression. Such depressions are quite common, and are often mistaken for manic depressive insanity. I myself have seen five cases of similar depression within the last four years.

After the analysis was completed the patient felt much relieved and grateful. I saw her a week later and there was not a trace of her former depression. She was cheerful and happy, and expressed her surprise at the sudden disappearance of her symptoms. She attributed it all to a mixture of rhubarb and soda which I gave her. She has had no attack of depression since then.

This short analysis teaches a number of things. First: There is a group of cases of periodic depression which do not belong to manic depressive insanity. They are anxiety hysterias based on somatic and psychosexual traumata. I am convinced that many cases that I have seen during my hospital service which were classified as manic depressive insanity and "depressions not sufficiently distinguished" belong to this category. Second: Freud's psychanalysis is, in my opinion, the only rational therapy for such cases, as it not only unravels the hidden mechanisms, but also removes the somatic sexual traumas, by correcting the abnormal sexual life. Third: The importance of dream analysis need hardly be emphasized. It is the *sine qua non* of the treatment.

A few words about examining the patient's psychosexual life. This, of course, presupposed a number of prerequisites. Not only must the physician himself be able to approach the subject without prudishness and lewdness, but he must, perforce, know something about psychosexuality. Unfortunately there are very few men in this country who take the subject seriously. Most physicians either ridicule or scorn those who have the courage to cope with sexual problems. For reasons known to themselves, but which we sometimes find in our psychanalytic work the word sexuality suffices to arouse their righteous indignation and to cause them to condemn everything connected with it. They seem to forget that besides the venereal diseases there are other sexual maladies requiring scientific treatment. Whatever is, has a reason, and it is the duty of every scientific man to view the cold facts honestly and fearlessly. Much unhappiness and misery would be eradicated if we would not leave these poor sexually distressed victims to the charlatans and quacks who not only rob them financially, but add to their misery and often drive them to suicide.

I have successfully treated by Freud's psychanalytic method cases of homosexuality, psychic impotence, sexual anesthesia in women, and many other so-called perversions, and my patients and I feel that distinct good has been done. To those who condemn us for recognizing the sexual life I can quote no fitter words than those of St. Augustine: "If what I have written scandalizes any prudish persons let them rather accuse the turpitude of their own thoughts than the words I have been obliged to use."

References

1. Freud: Selected Papers on Hysteria and Other Psychoneuroses, p. 149.

2. Freud: *L. c.*, p. 133.

3. Freud: *L. c.*, p. 141.

4. Freud: *L. c.*, p. 148.

5. Stekel: Nervöse Angstzustände und deren Behandlungen, Urban & Schwarzenberg, Wien, 1908.

6. Freud: The Interpretation of Dreams.

7. Freud: Sammlung kleiner Schriften zur Neurosenlehre, Zweite Folge, p. 159. Deuticke, Wein, 1909.

8. Jung: The Association Method. Translated by A. A. Brill, American Journal of Psychology, April, 1909. *Cf.* also Chap. V.

9. Jung: The Psychology of Dementia Præcox. Translated by Peterson and Brill, Journal of Nervous and Mental Dis. Pub. Co.

10 *Ibid.*, p. 141.

CHAPTER IV

THE COMPULSION NEUROSES (OBSESSIONS, DOUBTS, PHOBIAS)

Their Relation to the Sadistic Component and the Psychology of Love and Hatred

During the spring of 1909, the patient R., twenty-three years old, born in New York City, of Hebrew parentage, married, driver by occupation, applied for treatment in the neurological department of the Vanderbilt clinic. He was examined by Dr. C. Beling, who, after discussing the case with me, made the diagnosis "compulsion neurosis, probably paranoid," and referred the patient to the department of psychiatry to be treated by me.

R. was in excellent physical condition. There was nothing to attract one's attention to him anthropologically; his features were well formed and symmetrical, mentally he was alert and intelligent, answering questions readily and relevantly and his judgment and reasoning corresponded to his type—a bright, thoroughly Americanized young man of Russian-Jewish extraction.

According to the patient there was nothing to note about his family history. He was the only child and as far as he could judge there were no mental or nervous diseases in the family. His own life was not marked by any special events. He attended the public school up to the age of fourteen years and was a good student. After leaving school he worked and then peddled, first with his father and then alone in the neighboring farming districts. His present position he had obtained two years before. I will add here that upon entering somewhat deeper into my patient's symptom-complex I soon became convinced that I dealt with a case of compulsion neurosis and that there was nothing paranoid in it.

By compulsion neurosis in the Freudian sense we understand those cases which present obsessions, doubts and phobias and which are commonly called psychasthenias.

The patient sought treatment because for four years he had been annoyed by the thought that all the Jews would be killed by the Christians. To use his own words: "I have the idea that all Jews will be killed by Christians. I know the idea is foolish, but I cannot shake it off. It is always with me and at times is so strong that I almost believe it. I think that I will be killed because all Jews will be killed. I argue with myself about the impossibility of this idea, but I always come to the conclusion that although it is absurd it might happen and this naturally depresses me. I begin to worry and feel sorry for my poor father and I often cry over it."

What the patient himself thought strange was the fact that he had absolutely no reason for such thoughts. He never had any trouble with any Christian. On the contrary he could number many Christians among his friends. He had been employed by a Christian firm and was highly regarded and the one person with whom he had some differences was the only other Jew who was employed by the same firm. To my question he answered that on a few occasions he had thought of committing suicide. It came to him as a sort of a command: "You must die." But he argued that it would be useless to do it as the Christians would then cut up his body. He stated that the idea came on suddenly one day about four years before. It at first surprised and seemed strange to him, but he soon found that he could not rid himself of it. He had to think of it or of something referring to it. When asked to explain he said that he was always spinning fancies around it. He elaborated upon all sorts of abstruse questions in reference to it, *e.g.*, what kind of a world would it be after all the Jews were killed; what would Mrs. X. do; suppose Mr. Z. escapes, etc. As a result of all this he was very depressed, had no ambition and could take no interest in anything.

Besides these obsessions he complained of headaches and a peculiar "dull feeling" which came on from time to time and during which he could not think. He also stated that he was very often suspicious. He feared that some one would make remarks to him. This only occurred to him when he visited a public urinal.

We see then that the main feature of the case is the obsessive thinking. The only detail that would lead one to think of paranoia is the suspicion in public urinals.

As soon as the diagnosis was made I began to treat the patient by the psychanalytic method. Before entering into the analysis proper let us hear what Freud has to say on the mechanism of compulsion neurosis.

In his observation on the defense-neuropsychoses Freud describes the essence and mechanism of compulsion neurosis as follows:[1] "Sexual experiences of early childhood play the same part in the etiology of the compulsion neurosis as in hysteria but whereas the latter is characterized by passivity, the former is noted for its aggression or sexual activity. The essence of the compulsion neurosis may be expressed in the following formula: Obsessions are always transformed *reproaches* returning from repression which always refer to a pleasurably accomplished sexual action of childhood. The typical course of compulsion neurosis is as follows: The first period or the period of childish immorality contains the germs for the later neurosis. There is at first a sexual seduction which later makes the repression possible. This is followed by the actions of sexual aggressions against the other sex which later manifest themselves as actions of reproach. This period is brought to an end by the appearance of the—often self ripened—sexual maturity. A reproach then attaches itself to the memory of that pleasurable action and the connection with the initial experience of passivity makes it possible—only after conscious and recollected effort—to repress it and replace it by the primary symptom of the defense. The third period, that of apparent healthiness, but really of successful defense, begins with the symptoms of scrupulousness, shame and diffidence. The next period of the disease is characterized by the return of the repressed reminiscences, *i.e.*, by a failure of the defense. But the revived reminiscences and the reproaches formed from them never enter into consciousness unchanged. Instead, compromise formations between the repressed and repressing ideas become conscious as an obsession and obsessive affect and substitute the pathogenic memory in the conscious life. In the further course of the disease, depending on whether the memory content of the reproachful action alone forces an entrance into consciousness or whether it takes with it the accompanying reproaching affect, we may have two forms of the neurosis. The first represents the typical obsession, the content of which attracts the patient's attention. Only an indefinite displeasure is perceived as an affect, whereas for the content of the obsession the only suitable affect would be one of reproach. The second form of compulsion neurosis results if the repressed reproach and not the repressed content of memory forces a replacement in the conscious psychic sphere. The affect of the reproach can change itself into any other affect of displeasure, and if this occurs there is nothing to hinder the substituting affect from becoming conscious. Thus the reproach (of having performed in childhood some sexual actions) may be easily transformed into shame (lest someone becomes aware of it), into social fear (fearing punishment from others), into delusions of observation (fear of betraying those actions to others), into fear of temptation (justified distrust in one's own ability to resist), etc. Moreover, the memory content of the reproachful action may also be represented in consciousness, or it may be altogether concealed, which makes diagnosis very difficult. Many cases of the so-called "periodic neurasthenia" or "periodic melancholia" may be explained by compulsive affects.

Besides these compromise symptoms which signify a return of the repression and hence a failure of the originally achieved defense, the compulsion neurosis forms a series of other symptoms of a totally different origin.

The ego really tries to defend itself against those descendants of the initial repressed reminiscences and in this conflict of defense it produces symptoms which may be designated as "secondary defense." These are altogether protective measures which have performed good service in the struggle carried on against the obsession and the obsessing affects. If these helps in the conflict of the defense really succeed in repressing anew the symptoms of return, obtruding themselves on the ego, the compulsion then transmits itself on the protective measures themselves and produces a third form of the compulsion neurosis, the compulsive action. These are never primary. They never contain anything else but a defense, never an aggression. Despite their peculiarity they can always be fully explained by reduction to the compulsive reminiscences which they oppose.

The secondary defense of the obsessions can be brought about by a forcible deviation to other thoughts of possibly contrary content; hence in a case of success there is compulsive reasoning concerning abstract and transcendental subjects, because the repressed ideas always concern themselves with the sensuous, or the patient tries to become master of every compulsive idea through logical labor and by appealing to his conscious memory. This leads to compulsive thinking and examination and to doubting mania. The priority of the perception before the memory in these examinations at first induce and then force the patient to collect and preserve all objects with which he comes in contact. The secondary defense against the compulsive affects results in a greater number of defensive measures which are capable of being transformed into compulsive action. These can be grouped according to their tendency. We may have measures of penitence (irksome ceremonial and observation of numbers), of prevention (diverse phobias, superstitions, pedantry, aggravation of the primary symptom of scrupulousness), measures of fear of betrayal (collecting papers and shyness), and measures of becoming unconscious (dipsomania). Among these compulsive acts and impulses the phobias play the greatest part as limitations of the patient's existence."

Let us now return to our patient and see in how far he agrees with the description just read. Bearing in mind Freud's dictum that no neurosis is possible in a normal vita sexualis, I naturally made a thorough examination of the patient's psychosexual development. As usual in such examinations his answers were monosyllabic and evasive and all that I could elicit was that he was perfectly well sexually until the age of fifteen or sixteen years when he began to masturbate. He began to consort with women at eighteen years, but indulged rarely. He admitted that his marriage was not a happy one, but stated that his sexual life was normal. Previous to marriage he went through many conflicts. He was afraid that masturbation would drive him crazy and therefore stopped it, but he then began to suffer from frequent pollutions which worried him a good deal. He entertained the usual hypochondriacal ideas of the masturbator. He seemed to be unwilling to tell me anything else and I did not urge him. I was sure that there was abundant material and that he would tell it to me sooner or later. In the course of psychanalysis we often come to what seems a stone wall.

The patient has nothing to tell us and he does not dream. This is only a form of resistance which the experienced psychanalysist must know how to break.

As the character of a person represents the reaction formations of his latency period it is always wise to examine these reactions especially those that are accentuated, and as our patient seemed to be very shy—he never looked me in the face while talking—I asked him if he was unusually bashful. To my surprise he answered that bashfulness or shame was responsible for his obsession. He stated that he had been abnormally bashful and shy since he was twelve years old. This was especially noticeable when he was in the presence of women. A few years before he became acquainted with a young lady who invited him to call. He was very anxious to do so, but was too shy and bashful to accept her invitation. The following morning while half awake he noticed that he was not bashful. This gave him the idea that if he could remain in a half waking state he would not be bashful. He remained in this state for two days, when he suddenly began to think of Jews and Christians and later of the obsession. This half waking state was simply a secondary defense against a painful idea. The neuroses make prolific use of such mechanisms. Thus many dipsomanias are nothing but flights from consciousness or measures of becoming unconscious. I had occasion to analyze two female patients who were subject to screaming spells. They had to scream apparently without any provocation. Analysis showed that the screaming was merely a flight from a painful thought. With their screaming they drowned their inner painful and disagreeable voices. Many hysterical fainting spells show the same mechanism. Our patient merged into a semi-stuporous state not only to escape from the abnormal bashfulness, but from those thoughts which caused this reaction.

This revelation threw new light on the subject. From the nature of the obsession and the patient's extreme devotion to his parents, especially the father, I at once surmised that there was probably a strong repressed sadistic component and that the pronounced abnormal bashfulness could only be looked upon as a transformed reproach of sexual acts in childhood. On going more deeply into the infantile sexuality I discovered the following facts: R. was an only child and therefore received more than the usual amount of love from his parents.[2] He was idolized by both parents, especially by his mother with whom he slept almost constantly until the age of four years. This was favored by the fact that his father's business necessitated his remaining away from home for long periods. At that age something happened which changed his mother's attitude toward him. The patient attempted something of a sexual nature with a little girl with whom he played on the roof and was severly punished for it by the girl's and his own mother. The latter became very severe with him. She allowed him to sleep with her but kept him at a distance. He felt this very keenly and cried in silence, but said nothing. The mother instinctively reproached herself for the son's sexual prematurity. By giving him too much affection she awakened and kept alive his infantile sexuality which then incited him to attempt with the little girl what his own mother innocently permitted. The estrangement from his mother strengthened his attachment for his father and as the latter was rarely at home and made a great fuss over him whenever he returned that feeling continued for some time. The boy was very happy when his father returned and cried bitterly when he left home. It would seem that the latency period did not progress in the normal manner for the patient recalled many instances of sexual aggression and a homosexual experience with two adults. At the age of from six to seven years he was self-willed, wild and very revengeful. He evinced a special cruelty to animals and was happy when he could kill a bird or kick a cat. One of his favorite pastimes was to wring the necks of chickens or to stuff up their nasal openings with wax and hold their beaks until they suffocated.

We now come to the age of puberty. The patient recalled that at the age of nine years he was very inquisitive sexually and would look under girls' dresses whenever he could. At twelve years a man attempted to have sexual relations with him, but he refused. Soon thereafter he became shy and abnormally bashful. From twelve to fifteen years there were no sexual experiences to note. It may be called a deferred latency period. At fifteen he played with little girls and about the same time began to masturbate. When he was about sixteen, while peddling in the farming districts he began to exhibit in the presence of women. He claimed that this action gave him a "strange pleasant feeling." At the age of seventeen he began to practise active pederasty with a boy of thirteen which continued for about a year once every three weeks. At eighteen he began to consort with women, but with the exception of a few experiences he led a continent life until he was married at twenty-two years. Since the birth of his child he had practised coitus interruptus. His married life did not seem to influence his neurosis. He stated that he was especially annoyed by his obsession during the marriage ceremony, and that although the obsession was not so strong during the first year of his married life it soon resumed its former compulsiveness and constancy.

The facts that I have thus far obtained did not come out as smoothly as you might imagine. It was a constant struggle with enormous unconscious and conscious resistances, the overcoming of which required much effort and patience and, I might add, skill. But the patient soon became interested in the work and as the resistances were broken he spoke freely about his abnormal sexual life.

As has been stated before we make use of dream interpretation, for the dream is the via regia to the unconscious and at almost every session the patient brought me a few of his dreams. It was through these dreams that I discovered most of the details enumerated above. To show how the dream gives us information I will cite a dream which he brought about four months after the beginning of the analysis. It read as follows: "*I passed a store and saw a mad dog, a cat and a goat. A crowd was watching them. I said to somebody 'It is a wonder that they let that mad dog bite the horse'—just then a policeman began to shoot at the mad dog. He fired six shots, but missed it. The policeman then got in the window and was going to take the mad dog to the lock-up and it looked something like a horse and then it was a man.*" While still half asleep he said to himself "I must write that down for the doctor!"

To one who knows the language of the unconscious this dream tells many things. The appendix to the dream "I must write that down for the doctor" very often occurs in dreams in the course of psychanalysis and regularly corresponds to a great resistance to the confession involved in the dream and is frequently followed by the forgetting of the dream. It also means that the dreamer decided not to tell anything about it to the doctor. This was also confirmed by the crowd in the dream which signifies a secret. As the dreamer himself is always the principal actor in the dream I concluded that he must be concealed under the mad dog. This, too, is confirmed by the fact that the mad dog then becomes transformed into a man. But as the dog was also a horse there must be some community between the horse and the dog and the man. The nature of the dream shows that it is of a sexual nature.[3] When I asked him to tell me what the policeman brought to his mind he finally recalled a rather disagreeable reminiscence. At the age of fifteen he was in the habit of taking little girls on his lap and on the pretence of playing with them he masturbated. On one of these occasions in the Bronx Park he was suddenly detected by a policeman who ran after him and threatened to shoot him. Animals in dreams are usually sexual symbols and as he could give no associations I was convinced that there must have been something between him and the animals of a sexual nature. These are no arbitrary deductions, but they are based on psychological facts which all who are interested can find in Freud's "The Interpretation of Dreams." I did not hesitate to tell him my conclusions and after enormous resistance and great emotivity he admitted that he was guilty of bestiality with the horse, dog and sheep. This occurred while he was peddling in the farming districts between the ages of seventeen and eighteen. It was not a case of erotic zoophilia as he has not resorted to such practises since. It was simply a case of *faut de mieux* in a sexually hyperasthetic and very bashful boy.

In his "Three Contributions to the Sexual Theory" Freud states that the constitutional sexual predisposition of the child is more irregularly multifarious than one would expect; that it deserves to be called "polymorphous perverse" and that from this predisposition the so-called normal behavior of the sexual functions results through the repression of certain partial impulses and components of the infantile predisposition, and through the subordination of the rest under the primacy of the genital zones for the service of the function of procreation. The perversions correspond to a disturbance of this connection due to a superior compulsive-like development of some of the partial impulses, while the neurosis could be traced to a marked repression of the libidinous strivings. Without going into any detailed comparisons, I will simply state that a study of our patient's psychosexual life agrees in every particular with what I have just quoted from Freud. Let us now see how this corresponds with the patient's compulsive idea.

When I first heard the principal obsession, viz., that all the Jews will be killed by the Christians, I was, perforce, reminded of such personages as Catherine de Medici and Gil de Rais; I was struck by the idea of such unheard of wholesale slaughter, and remembering that the symptom represents the whole or a partial sexual manifestation of the patient from the sources of the normal or perverse partial impulses of sexuality, I naturally thought that there must be a marked sadistic component in the patient's psychosexuality. As I have shown above, my assumption was fully confirmed. Further investigations of the causes of the obsession in mature life brought out the fact that it appeared suddenly at about the age of twenty while the patient was seriously thinking of marrying, and just after getting over an unhappy love affair. This amour was with the daughter of a farmer whose acquaintance he made while traveling near her home. He was very fond of the girl and would have married her but for his father who would not hear of his marrying a Christian. His father played a peculiar part in R.'s life. There was a constant struggle of the two contrary feelings of love and hatred. Paradoxical as it may seem, he hated him as intensely as he loved him. The continued existence of such contrasts is possible only under special psychic determination and with the help of the unconscious state. We know that the contrasting feelings of love and hatred can be readily entertained in reference to indifferent persons. Thus, a clerk may think that his superior is an excellent executive man, but an unscrupulous lawyer. But when it concerns some one nearer to us, let us say a wife or parent, we strive for a single feeling and we therefore overlook the faults which may provoke displeasure. But the love does not extinguish the hatred. It merely represses it into the unconscious where it is kept from destruction and may even grow in intensity.[4] The determination of this peculiar constellation of love lies in the separation of these contrasting feelings and a repression of one—usually the hatred—at a very early age. As a preliminary explanation of the compulsion neurosis, Freud states that the sadistic component of love was especially strongly developed constitutionally in those cases of unconscious hatred and for that reason they were subjected to a premature and thorough suppression. The phenomena of the neurosis, then, take their origin on the one hand from the conscious attachment which comes to the surface through reaction and on the other hand from the unconscious sadism in operation. If we review the patient's relation to his father we find that at an early age he was, as it were, his rival. Whenever the father was home he had to renounce many pleasures, such as sleeping with his mother. Later on when his mother changed her attitude toward him he became very attached to his father, but he often had occasion to hate him because he often punished him. As he grew older these feelings were intensified by the fact that his father was an orthodox Jew and he wanted to be an American. He was ashamed to be seen with his father because the street urchins made derogatory remarks about him. They called him Jew and Sheeny. He himself often applied the same epithets to him, which was naturally followed by a reproach and an outburst of affection. When his father opposed his marriage with the Christian the old rivalry was revived. His father again stood in his way of attaining his sexual object. Just as he kept him away from his mother during childhood so he now prevented him from marrying. His feeling for the girl was also characterized by the contrasts of love and hatred, but whereas this was largely a conscious perception, his former intense conscious hostility toward his father escaped him long ago and could only be brought to consciousness in the face of the most violent resistance. This was especially favored by his long abstinence and recent love which thus helped to enhance his libido and to take up again the old struggle against the authority of the father. We may say that the repression of the infantile hatred toward his father gave rise to all further happenings of the neurosis. While he was wavering between his father and his beloved and escaped from conscious reflection by merging into a semi-stuperous state, he was one day attracted by the big red head lines of a newspaper about the massacre of the Jews in Russia. As his father was a Russian Jew a thought something like the following suddenly flashed through his mind: "If my father were only there!" which may be completed "he would be killed and I could marry a Christian;" but this conscious perception was naturally at once suppressed. A few days later he began to compare notes about Jews and Christians which finally developed into the obsession "All Jews will be killed by Christians." In other words the whole process followed the well-known mechanism of projection, *i.e.*, an inner perception is suppressed and as a substitute its content comes into consciousness as a perception from without after it has undergone some distortion. The distortions are effected in the same way as in dreams, *i.e.*, by substitution, displacement, inversion, ellipses, etc. Here it was not a real distortion, but rather a generalization which is a common mechanism of obsessions.[5]

After this analysis the obsession from which the patient

had suffered for about four years and which had caused him untold misery soon disappeared. The treatment lasted for about four months, during which I saw the patient at first three times a week, then twice and once a week. We usually spent an hour at each session. The patient was by no means cured. There was still much to be done. Thus his homosexual component had to be dealt with.* After eight months treatment I discharged him as cured. Since then he has become more ambitious. He gave up his position as driver and is now the owner of a well paying business.

The analysis of this case fully confirms Freud's assertion that a special aggressive activity in childhood is characteristic of the later compulsion neurosis. This activity manifests itself preponderately in an intensive occupation with the desire for looking and knowing. The rich and active emotional life of childhood helps to develop profusely the feelings of love and hatred toward parents, or sisters and brothers, which, in addition to the curiosity concerning sex and birth, forms the central complex of the neurosis. One always finds in the symptom formation of compulsion neurosis a continuous struggle between love and hatred for the same person, and as we said above such feeling is only possible under special psychic determinations.

However, whenever an intensive love is confronted by just as strong a hatred there always results a partial paralysis of volition. It is an inability to form decisions in all those actions for which love forms the motive power.

* Analysis showed that his suspicion in public urinals was due to a repressed wish to exhibit in order to attract those near him.

This indecision does not confine itself long to one group but becomes diffused over all actions by the familiar mechanism of displacement.

This gives rise to the predominance of compulsion and doubt as we find them in the psychic life of compulsive neurotics. "Doubt corresponds to the inner perception of the indecision, which in consequence of the inhibition of love through hatred usurps every intentional action of the patient."[6] It is really the doubt about love, which should be the most certain of all things subjective, which spreads on everything else and then becomes displaced on the most indifferent trifles. He who doubts his love must also doubt everything of lesser importance. A few years ago I was consulted by a man of fifty-six years who was obsessed with the idea that he was not fit for the position he occupied. He stated that he was not sure of his actions, that no matter what he did he imagined was wrong, and that he really made many business mistakes. He resigned his position as manager of a big business concern, but after examining everything the officers of the company were satisfied that he made no mistakes at all and insisted upon his remaining with them. I myself spoke with a member of the firm who told me that during his thirty years service there had been no complaints against him. The patient admitted that he was quite capable of filling his office up to a few months before but that since then he had been doubting the correctness of his business transactions. In brief it was a typical case of doubting mania.

The analysis revealed the following facts: The neurosis became manifest when he was about to marry a young woman who was twenty-two years his junior. He at first worried over the fact that he would not be able to "make good" as a husband, because he believed himself to be sexually impotent. This doubt then became generalized and displaced to all his business transaction. Long before he consulted me he no longer thought of his sexual impotence but occupied himself constantly with absurd questions concerning legitimate business affairs.

The same doubt which produces uncertainty and leads to continued repetition in the protective measures, in order to drive away uncertainty, finally brings it about that these protective acts become just as impossible of accomplishment as the originally inhibited decision of love. Thus a patient recommended to me by Dr. Pierce Bailey of New York was in the habit of praying for an hour and sometimes even longer before retiring. His father stated that he could not be stopped and that he usually fell asleep while praying on his knees. This patient was not very religious. He told me that his prayers were constantly interrupted by extraneous blasphemous thoughts which usually repeated the opposite of what he was praying for. Investigation showed that his prayers were usually offered for those who played the leading part in his neurosis and that the fancies obtruding themselves contained the opposite impulse of that which the prayer was to ward off.

The compulsion, however, is an attempted compensation for the doubt and a correction for the unbearable state of inhibition as evidenced by the doubt. If any of the inhibited resolutions is finally decided upon, it must be brought to completion. To be sure it is no longer the original one, but its dammed in energy will not abandon the opportunity of finding an outlet through the substitutive action. It therefore manifests itself in commands and prohibitions depending on whether the loved or the hostile impulse occupies the path of discharge. If the obsessive command cannot be brought to execution it produces an unbearable tension which is perceived as marked anxiety.

These are some of the deeper mechanisms of compulsion neurosis. I realize that some may find them somewhat too complicated to follow, but the only way of obviating these difficulties is close study and personal experience.

References

1. Selected papers on Hysteria, p. 155.
2. *Cf.* Chap. X on The Only Child.
3. *Cf.* Chap. III.
4. Jahrb. f. Psychoanal. u. Psychopath. Forschungen, Vol. I,p. 375.
5. *L. c.*, p. 419.
6. *L. c.*, p. 416.

CHAPTER V

PSYCHANALYSIS AND THE PSYCHOSES

The Work of the Zurich School—the Association Experiment—Complex Theory—Mechanism of Delusions and Hallucinations

The conclusions reached by Freud as expressed in the theories of the psychoneuroses, dreams and the psychopathology of everyday life were fully confirmed by the Zurich school after a thorough investigation on the basis of experimental psychology. Stimulated by Bleuler, Jung and Riklin[1] collected a large number of associations from normal persons with the intention of finding out, first, whether there existed any regularity in the reactions and, second, whether there were definite reaction types. They soon discovered that the process of association is a very flighty and variable psychic process and that it is beyond the limits of objective control. They also found that attention plays the greatest part in the process of association. Although it directs and modifies the associative process it can nevertheless be most readily controlled experimentally. They therefore decided to investigate experimentally the following questions: 1. The laws of fluctuation in associations in the normal, and 2. the direct effects of attention on the process of association, especially whether the validity of association relatively diminishes with the distance from the fixation point of consciousness.

They examined many educated and uneducated persons by giving them a hundred stimulus words and noting the reactions. The reaction time was measured with a one-fifth second stop watch. The second series of experiments consisted of 100 associations with internal distraction. The third series consisted of 100 associations taken during external distraction by means of a metronome. The results obtained from 12,400 associations showed many interesting facts of which only few will interest us here.

After classifying the associations it was found that there was a distinct fluctuation in the numerical relations of single individuals. The main reason for this was the intensity of attention. That accounted for the fact that some reacted with inner and others with outer associations. It was found, for example, that although every person had manifold qualities of associations at his disposal, the reactions elicited nevertheless depended on the degree of attention evoked by the stimulus words. Thus, whenever the test person was distracted he always reacted with outer and sound association rather than with inner associations, *i.e.*, he followed the lines of least resistance and reacted with habitual and easy speech combinations. Jung concluded that whenever there is a disturbance of attention one must expect shallow reaction types or sound associations and, conversely, whenever one finds sound associations he must presuppose a disturbance of attention.

Without entering into the theoretical part of associations in general I will now show the practical side of the work as it is applied in the Clinic of Psychiatry at Zurich.

One hundred words are usually employed for analytic and diagnostic purposes. They are designated as test words and were selected and arranged in a manner to strike almost all of the common complexes. The test words are printed in rows with enough side space for the test person's answers or reactions. The experiment is carried out with the test person sitting in front of the physician who calls out each word in a loud and clear voice, measuring at the same time with a one-fifth of a second stop watch the time elapsing between the utterance of the test word and the reaction or the answer from the test person. The average reaction time is generally taken as 2.4 seconds. Before the experiment is begun the test person is instructed to pay attention to the test words and answer as quickly as possible the first word that comes to his mind. The answers, as well as the reaction time, are carefully noted and after the whole list has been gone through, the stimulus words are repeated and the patient is asked to reproduce the original answers which are again noted. Depending on the case in question some special words may be inserted, but as a rule the following 100 words are used:

1. head
2. green
3. water
4. to sing
5. dead
6. long
7. ship
8. to pay
9. window
10. friendly
11. to cook
12. to ask
13. cold
14. stem
15. to dance
16. village
17. lake
18. sick
19. pride
20. table
21. ink
22. angry
23. needle
24. to swim
25. voyage
26. blue
27. lamp
28. to sin
29. bread
30. rich
31. tree
32. to prick
33. pity
34. yellow
35. mountain
36. to die
37. salt
38. new
39. custom

40. to pray
41. money
42. foolish
43. pamphlet
44. despise
45. finger
46. expensive
47. bird
48. to fall
49. book
50. unjust
51. frog
52. to part
53. hunger
54. white
55. child
56. to take care
57. lead pencil
58. sad
59. plum
60. to marry
61. house
62. dear
63. glass
64. to quarrel
65. fur
66. big
67. carrot
68. to paint
69. part
70. old
71. flower
72. to beat
73. box
74. wild
75. family
76. to wash
77. cow
78. friend
79. luck
80. lie
81. deportment
82. narrow
83. brother
84. to fear
85. stork
86. false
87. anxiety
88. to kiss
89. bride
90. pure
91. door
92. to choose
93. hay
94. contented
95. ridicule
96. to sleep
97. month
98. nice
99. woman
100. to abuse

Now it would seem that any intelligent person could give a fluent answer to any of these words but one soon becomes convinced that such is not the case. As one proceeds with the experiment he finds that not all stimulus words are reacted to with the same smoothness and facility. In his "Association method"[2] Jung shows that all apparently adventitious mistakes in the association experiment have a definite reason and that contrary to the belief of the test person his answers are not at all arbitrary, but generally betray his inmost secrets. Hence whenever we find any impediments in the experiment such as a prolonged reaction time, a lack of or a faulty reaction, a repetition of the stimulus words or a failure of reproduction we have a *complex indicator*. That is, the mistake indicates that the stimulus word has touched a complex* and thus retarded or completely inhibited the reaction.

The value of this experiment is quite obvious. Whereas the patient may refuse to enter into conversation about his morbid productions he is quite willing to cooperate in the experiment. He sees no harm in answering the first word evoked by the stimulus as he is entirely unaware of its import. Some think it is a "sort of game" which has no bearing on their condition. But as soon as a few complexes are found and the association correctly interpreted the patient readily recognizes the superiority of the examiner and generally talks freely. As I will show later this is not as simple as it may seem. To illustrate the actual work I will cite the following cases:

Case I.—I. S., æt. thirty-nine, single, bank official, was transferred to the psychiatric clinic of Zurich, November 16, 1907, from the Bohemian asylum of D. where he had been for about four months. From the abstract we learned that the patient went through an acute attack lasting only a few weeks. He was markedly confused and hallucinatory, but gradually improved. He had not, however, regained any insight into his condition and still entertained numerous false ideas.

On admission he was orderly and well behaved. He seemed to take a lively interest in things, but was inclined to be seclusive and uncommunicative. When drawn into conversation he gave a fair account of his experiences, but now and then he only vaguely intimated things, absolutely refusing to enter into details. His orientation was perfect, no hallucinations of any kind could be elicited, though he showed no insight into his condition. Physically, besides diminished knee-jerks, nothing abnormal could be found. He gave a fluent account of his *vita anteacta* and only here and there was it necessary to question him.

* The word is used in the sense designated by the Zurich school, *i.e.*, as a complex of ideas of marked emotional accentuation which was split off from consciousness and repressed into the unconscious.

He stated that he was born in W. near Zurich. His mother was an invalid for years. She suffered from some "nervous trouble" and died when he was about ten years old. His father, an octogenarian, was still living. He knew nothing about the other members of his family for since his eleventh year he had been brought up among strangers. Up to his sixteenth year he was under the guidance of a clergyman who brought him up very religiously. He attended school up to his seventeenth year when he began his business career and since his twentieth year he had worked in the bank of B. He saw his father quite frequently up to 1903 when there was a disagreement between them ending in a complete estrangement. When asked about the cause of this quarrel he at first refused to speak of it, but on being urged he said: "The last time my father was in B. I told him that I would like to marry my landlady, a widow, in whose house I lived for more than seven years. He strongly objected and threatened to disown me should I disobey him. He also upbraided me for my mode of living. He is very religious and antisemitic while I was an agnostic and worked among Jews for eighteen years. I reminded him that I was old enough to follow my own inclinations and so we parted. Since then I have written to him a number of times, but all my letters have been returned to me."

His psychosis he described as follows: "I was always well until the beginning of February, when I suddenly became thoughtful. I did not sleep well and was very nervous. On February 3, 1907, at 7 P. M., I was alone in my room when I began to feel a strange power influencing me. I felt ecstatic, but I knew that there was something peculiar in me. It was like an electric magnetic power or ether. It suddenly forced me down on the floor on my left knee. My hands were pressed together in an attitude of prayer and with great force I cried out: 'Lord, have mercy on suffering humanity.' I spoke with a stentorian voice like a preacher. I repeated the 'Our Father' hundreds of times. I felt an influence of the Egyptian gods Isis and Osiris. I was also forced to repeat numerous times 'Am I Parsifal, the guileless fool?' (Parsifal reinster Thor). This state continued for seventy-two hours during which I did not sleep at all. I also imagined that I was very wealthy. The whole thing was like a colossal suggestive influence and the Jews played some part in it. After four days I got out of bed and took a walk which refreshed me, but I caught a cold which continued for six weeks. During that time I was under the magic of a peculiar suggestive inspiration in which the Jews played a great part."

Asked whether he heard voices talking to him he stated that he heard none during the first crisis. "It was only a magnetic suggestive force." Continuing, he said: "I then wrote a letter to my firm with whom I had been for eighteen years, telling them that my present views did not permit me to work for a Jewish firm. Following an inspiration I went to Lucarno where I remained until April 5. I then returned to B. and in order to recover completely I went to a country place near the sea where I remained for five weeks. In June I went to see my father, who lived in K., Bohemia, but was not permitted to see him as his doctor forbade it, saying he was too sick. I could not believe that the doctor told me the truth. It was certainly remarkable that my old father should estrange himself in such a manner from his only son. At the end of June I was offered a position in Munich, but when I arrived there I found that the head of the firm was a Jew so I refused it. On July 14, a letter sent to my father was returned marked 'Moved. Address unknown.' I again became excited and felt the peculiar suggestive inspirations. Such inspirations were never in me before and probably had their reasons. . . . . . I again went to K., arriving there on July 16. My father's residence was locked and the neighbors told me that he had moved to D. I decided to follow up my investigations the next morning, but 'Man proposes and God disposes.' I passed a fearful night. I was continually under influences. I dreamed that I climbed a high mountain or mountains and all of a sudden I became 'like nailed' and I could not move any further. I was afraid of falling and was extremely terrified. At dawn I arose and decided to take a walk in the forest, but no sooner did I leave the hotel when I suddenly heard a voice in my ears. I looked about alarmed, but saw no one. The voice asked me peculiar questions and gave still stranger commands. It was something like telepathy. I almost lost my mind. I noticed two policemen and I appealed to them for protection. They took me to the police station and then I only faintly recollect being taken to a hospital in a cab. I was in an unconscious, peculiar, feverish state. I heard voices constantly, but they were very indistinct. I saw silhouettes like bluish angelic forms. I saw my father. He was God and I was the Son, and Superintendent R. was the Holy Ghost. I was in that condition for about one week and then I recovered my senses. They then sent me to the asylum in D. and on November 16 I was transferred here."

The last part of the patient's statements concurs with the hospital records from D. He finished by paraphrasing Hamlet, "There are more things in heaven and earth, doctor, than are dreamt of in your psychiatry."

An attempt was made to have the patient explain some of the individual points, but he became diplomatic and suspicious, saying that he had told everything to the best of his ability and that he really could not remember any more. Besides he was sure that no doctor could understand this or explain it to him, that he was perfectly well now and only wished to be discharged so that he might go and see his old father. When asked what he thought of the whole affair he said that he was sure the whole thing was something divine and supernatural and also implied that he understood it all. No amount of urging, however, could induce him to enter deeper into the question.

In the ward, besides his seclusiveness, nothing abnormal could be noticed. He spent most of his time in reading. He also wrote numerous letters to his father and friends, telling them about his strange experiences, and assuring them that he was now completely changed and perfectly well both physically and mentally. During my visits he was always affable, but, except concerning his discharge, he evinced no desire to enter into conversation. When an attempt was made to question him he immediately stated "that it was time wasted and that he had told me all he knew," and always ended with his preferred quotation, mentioned above, "There are many things, doctor, etc." Only on a few occasions was it possible to induce him to explain some of the details.

This condition remained essentially unchanged for more than two months when he was discharged: Diagnosis, dementia præcox.

For those who work up their cases on a Kraepelin-Wernicke basis the problem, if not solved, is finished. To be sure the case could be elaborated upon. A detailed description of the various incidents could be given, but no matter how extensive and detailed it might be made, if we followed Kraepelin the personal factors would be very meagerly, if at all, considered. Indeed, Kraepelin in all his works, gives very accurate and faithful descriptions of his cases, but he does not go beyond that. It makes no difference what the nature of a special case may be so long as it fulfils certain conditions as regards the emotional status, morbid perceptions, delusions, mannerisms, etc. In other words Kraepelin totally ignores individual psychology.

However, both on the continent and in this country the tendency now is to pay more attention to individual psychology. Instigated by the valuable discoveries of Freud, the Zurich school took up the problem and the results, as every one knows, are most gratifying. In this country A. Meyer and August Hoch approached the problem from a somewhat different standpoint but came to essentially the same conclusions, namely, that attention must be paid to the actual cases and that a mere general description does not suffice. The works of Bleuler, Jung, Riklin and others show how effete and soulless the old routine methods of description appear in comparison to the very interesting psychanalytic methods where one finds a definite relation between cause and effect. In making these statements I do not wish to detract in any way from the great merits of Kraepelin whose epoch-making works in modern psychiatry everyone duly recognizes; but the superiority of Kraepelin's methods over those of his predecessors only serves to emphasize their deficiencies when compared to the psychanalytic methods.

As aforesaid it was impossible to draw the patient into ordinary conversation for any length of time, so that I started by taking his associations and then analyzed them. The following associations are given:

Stimulus Word	*Reaction*	*Time**	*Reproduction*
1. Coal	Burning Material	3.4	X†
2. Moderate	Temperance	4.2	Wine Beer
3. Song	Singing Club	3.6	X
4. To Suppose	To Doubt	5.2	Religion
5. Pain	Body	2.6	Physical Pain
6. Lazy	Schoolboy	4.2	Urchin
7. Moon	Heaven	3.6	Venus
8. To Laugh	Society	2.6	X
9. Coffee	Drink	4.4	Coffee Table
10. Broad	Board	2.4	X

Ass. 1, "coal-burning material" shows a long reaction time. This is frequently seen in the beginning of the experiment. On analysis it recalls many reminiscences of his youth when he lived in the coal regions of B. Ass. 2, "moderate—temperance—wine, beer" refers to his complex of drink. At the age of twenty-five he drank much beer, his father often spoke to him about moderation. Ass. 3, "song—singing club," recalls the singing club of B. which patient often visited, it especially recalls a dirge which he once heard and this recalls his dead sweetheart. Ass. 4, "to suppose—to doubt—religion" refers to the complex of religion. He supposed that there was no God and he doubted all religion, but now he is quite convinced that the contrary is true. Ass. 5, "pain—body—physical pain" refers to rheumatic pain to which he is subject, but mainly to the pains caused by his father's behavior in ignoring him. Ass. 6, "Lazy—schoolboy—urchin" refers to the seven-year-old son of the widow with whom he boarded. Patient showed numerous resistances and

* The time is indicated in seconds.

† X = correct reproduction.

obstructions and finally refused to continue with this association. Ass. 7, "moon—heaven—Venus." Asked to explain this strange association he said: "On March 28 I awoke during the night and there was a beautiful moon. I had a suggestive dream. I thought that it could be possible to walk on the water and be born like Venus was." He then refused to continue, but after many obstructions and inhibitions he said that by water he means the Atlantic and Venus refers to his sweetheart who died in America. The day before, he saw a picture in the Berliner Illustrierte Zeitung of a newly discovered "sea-people" with webbed fingers and toes who either barked or prayed to the moon. Ass. 9, "coffee—drink—coffee table" recalls a friend in Guatemala, a coffee planter, who just married a Swiss girl and this recalls his "first and only sweetheart" who married in America. This may also refer to his drinking complex. Ass. 10, "broad-board" recalls a broad tree trunk, broad breast . . . . . (sudden obstruction).

Stimulus Word	*Reaction*	*Time*	*Reproduction*
11. Air	Ether	3.4	Body
12. To frighten	Oh terror	4.2	To collapse
13. Plate	Table	2.0	X
14. Tired	Walk	3.2	X
15. Intention	Resolution	6.0	Determination of will
16. To fly	Bird	1.8	X
17. Eye	Head	4.8	Angel
18. Fruit	Vegetable	3.0	X
20. To work	Office	2.2	X
21. To sail	Ocean	4.8	X
22. Modest	Virtue	7.4	Quality
23. Soil	Earth	3.2	X
24. To whistle	Schoolboy	2.2	X

Ass. 11, "air—ether—body" refers to ether which filled his body during his first attack. Ass. 12, "to frighten—oh terror—to collapse" is explained as follows: "When I first heard the voices in K. I became so terrified that I almost collapsed. It was so real, as though some one was near me. I remained 'like nailed.' Then I called out 'who talks to me and what is your name?' The voice replied 'water, drink water.'" (See Ass. 7.) It was so terrible, especially after the frightful night, I did not sleep at all during that night. I thought some one was in the room and I looked under the bed, but I found no one. I also dreamed of climbing mountains. I arose at 5.30 and then a suggestive thought almost like a voice said: 'Jump from the fourth floor window and if you believe you will rise unharmed.' Then another suggestion said 'How can you do it, you are only a sinner' and then I left the hotel. Ass. 14, "intention—resolution—determination of will" is explained as follows: "Between 1890 and 1895 I drank considerably. Then I formed a resolution not to drink and I was a total abstainer until 1899 when I was operated upon for hemorrhoids. Since then I drank moderately. I also resolved never to marry. When I was twenty-two I had a sweetheart, a very pretty girl, Marie Biere. I was very anxious to marry her, but my father objected to it, saying that I was only a young fool, etc. In 1887 she went to America, to Pittsburgh, Pa., but before going we promised to be true to each other. In 1888 I heard she married a Swiss in Pittsburgh. I was very dejected. It was my first real and true love. I had many sweethearts after that, but I never loved another woman. I then went to Paris and just cast myself into the whirl so as to forget everything and I finally forgot her. In 1891 I heard she died." (While reciting this the patient became very emotional). Ass. 17, "eye—head—angel" recalls his father's head, "he has a wonderful eye like Bismark—it is God's eye." (He has only one eye). (In his delirium his father was God, etc., see above.) Ass. 21, "sail—ocean" shows a very long reaction time. He thinks of America where he was so very anxious to go, but his father objected. Ass. 22, "modest—virtue—quality" cannot be explained. He began to speak of modest women but suddenly stopped. It probably has some erotic sense.* Ass. 23, "soil—earth" shows a long reaction time due to a perseveration of former reaction; probably refers to dream about birth of Venus. Ass. 24, "whistle—schoolboy" is another reference to the boy mentioned in Ass. 6; he showed many obstructions and finally asked not to be questioned about it. Ass. 25, "aim—intention" is a perseveration of the former—he says "Everything has its reasons, dress is only to cover the body"—probably some erotic complex.

Stimulus Word	*Reaction*	*Time*	*Reproduction*
26. Hat	Summer	3.4	X
27. Hand	Body	2.6	God's hand
28. To wake	In bed	2.4	To get out of bed
29. Apple	You have I believe	3.8	Fruit tree vegetables
30. Evil	Quality	2.6	X
31. Mouth	Head	3.6	Boy
32. To drink	Thirst	3.4	An inn
33. Bed	To sleep	2.6	X
34. Pretty	Pretty girl	4.4	Beer
35. Danger	Mountain	5.0	Mountain fall

* The word is used in its original Greek sense, as anything appertaining to love—eros.

Stimnlus Word	*Reaction*	*Time*	*Reproduction*
36. To visit	Friends	3.0	X
37. Laborer	Mason	2.2	X
38. High	Mountain	2.6	X
39. Axe	Instrument	2.4	Carpenter
40. To observe	Adjective	4.0	School

Ass. 27, "hand—body—God's hand" is not explained, but it probably refers to his religious complex. Ass. 28, "to wake—in bed—to get out of bed" refers to expression "wide awake boy" and this again recalls the son of his landlady (obstruction emotivity). Ass., 29 "apple—you have I believe—fruit tree vegetables" is a perseveration of former reaction, or may have an erotic sense—he is unable "to explain it." Ass. 30, "evil—quality" evokes "bad boy" meaning the landlady's boy as does the following Ass. 31, "mouth—head—boy" which he explains as "human mouth connected with chewing, eating, etc."—mother's mouth—"I have never done such dirty things." Asked to explain what he means he at first refused to continue and on being urged he said "I think of the scenes that I witnessed in Paris." This was followed by a sudden outburst of excitement. He jumped up and talked very excitedly. He saw no reason why he should be forced to talk of such dirty things, that he never would think of it if not for the experiments, etc. He was so irritable that the analysis had to be stopped for a week. Ass. 32, "drink—thirst—inn" refers to his alcoholic complex. Ass. 34, "pretty—pretty girl—beer" refers to his sweetheart whose name was Biere. Ass. 35, "danger—mountain—mountain fall" refers to his dreams of mountain climbing. He also stated that he was once in danger of falling off a steep mountain and was only saved by the timely arrival of a mountain guide. Ass. 38, "high—mountain" again refers to his mountain climbing and also to the frightful dreams about climbing at the onset of the second crisis. Ass 40, "to observe—adjective—school" refers again to the schoolboy and, as usual, the patient could not "explain it."

Stimulus Word	*Reaction*	*Time*	*Reproduction*
41. Road	I also think of a lawn	4.0	Forest
42. Round	Globe	2.2	X
43. Blood	Operation	5.2	Knight
44. To state	School	4.2	Schoolboy
45. Attention	da-danger	4.8	Quality
46. Gay	Society	3.2	X
47. Market	Stock market	4.2	Money
48. To forget	Time	5.4	Love
49. Drum	Carnival	3.6	X
50. Free	Air	4.8	X

Ass. 41, "road—I also think of a lawn-forest" refers to the morning of his second attack when he arose early to go into the forest. Ass. 43, "blood—operation—knight" the patient states that in 1899 he underwent an operation for hemorrhoids during which he lost much blood. It also recalls the blood of the grail referred to in Parsifal. From blood he also goes to the word "blutt" which means naked and this recalls a dream fragment about arms and breasts which he had on the night of July 16. Ass. 44, "to state—school—schoolboy" refers again to his landlady's boy. Ass. 45, "attention—da-danger—quality" refers to his last attack when the voices addressed him. Ass. 47, "market—stock market—money" refers to his trade complex. Ass. 48, "to forget—time—love" he explained as follows: "love is in time forgotten." Ass. 50, "free—air" refers to his confinement.

Stimulus Word	*Reaction*	*Time*	*Reproduction*
51. Religion	The living word	4.2	Thomas
52. Jews	Deutches Volksblatt	3.4	Rich
53. Isis	Osiris	3.0	Banker
54. Widow	Wehrli	2.6	X
55. Parsifal	Knight	4.0	Guileless fool
56. Father	Love	2.8	X

Ass. 51, "religion—the living word—Thomas" was explained as follows: "Despite my being brought up religiously I became a free-thinker and for years I never thought of religion. I scoffed at everything. I was the real 'doubting Thomas.' I studied Nietzsche and especially Max Stirner, whose last book 'Der Einzige u. sein Eigentum (The Ego and His Own)' has the motto, 'All things are nothing with me.' It is a very dangerous book. But all my ideas and plans have been crushed because I could not conceive the real and holy religion. What happened to me within the last year is a sign sent from above, 'the true living word' which forces me to seek God. I have still something of the 'doubting Thomas,' but it will soon disappear." Ass. 52, "Jews—Deutsches Volksblatt—rich." Patient denied bearing any animosity against Jews. He worked eighteen years with Jews and always got along very nicely with them. "They are very nice rich people," he said, but for some reason which he is unable to explain he was a constant subscriber to the Deutsches Volksblatt, which he claims is an antisemitic journal. Ass. 53, "Isis—Osiris—banker" refers to Mr. Osiris, a very wealthy banker in Basel, who died before the patient's first attack. The patient says that he now recalls that during the first attack he had the idea that this banker left him 30,000,000 francs. Some one told him so. He denies ever having had any relations with Mr. Osiris. Osiris is a contiguous association of Isis. Ass. 54, "widow—Wehrli" refers to Mrs. Wehrli, his landlady, with whom he boarded for seven years. He stated that he really did not love her, but he liked her and seriously thought of marrying her. In 1903 he spoke about it to his father who objected to it. After Christmas, 1907, he resolved to save money and then marry her, but since the last attack he gave up the idea. Ass. 55, "Parsifal—knight—guileless fool" refers to Parsifal as depicted in Wagner's opera, where he is named the guileless fool. Patient seemed to identify himself with the knight, but did not fully explain it. Like Parsifal he had to undergo many vicissitudes before recognizing the true religion. But we shall return to this later. Ass. 56, "father—love" is not fully explained. Patient said: "There were times during which I almost hated my father, but now I am very much concerned about him and am very anxious to see him."

One hundred and fifty associations have been taken from the patient, but the given associations are sufficient for the explanation of the principal complexes and to give us a fair understanding of the symptomatic ideogenesis. The main characteristics of the associations are the long reaction times and faulty reproductions. As we have said above the average reaction time of persons of his type is taken as 2.4 seconds. In the associations given about 84 per cent. are above the normal reaction time and only about 43 per cent. of the reactions are correctly reproduced. These are the so-called complex-indicators and wherever they occur are taken as signs of complex constellations.

The stimulus word either consciously or unconsciously touched the complex and this evoked the intervention of a presentation of strong feeling tone. This always happens in normal and neurotic individuals and Jung has shown that the same holds true in Dementia Præcox.

When we examine the nature of the associations we find that sixteen (3, 7, 9, 15, 21, 22, 23, 25, 29, 31, 34, 35, 45, 53, 54, 58) belong to the erotic complex, seven (4, 11, 12, 27, 43, 51, 52) to the complex of religion and six (6, 24, 28, 30, 31, 40) directly concern the "boy." Unfortunately the last associations were not satisfactorily explained by the patient. Judging from the very strong repression which dominated them we are quite certain that they play a great part in the patient's psyche. Two suppositions should be kept in mind:

(1) Patient may be the father of the boy.

(2) There may have been some homosexual relations between them. In favor of (1) is the fact that he boarded for more than seven years with the boy's mother (the boy was about seven years old). A number of letters exchanged between the patient and his landlady point to that. If he is not his son there probably was some homosexual relation between them as shown by Ass. 31. We are therefore perfectly justified in adding these six associations to the erotic which gives a total of twenty-two. The religious complexes, too, are intimately connected with the erotic.

Bearing this in mind we can form an idea of the part played by the erotic in the patient's psyche. We can say that almost all his psychical components when thoroughly analyzed show some relation to it. This may seem peculiar, but it is not at all unusual, it is found in all psychoneuroses as well as in the normal. According to Freud all so-called day dreams in women are of an erotic nature.[3] In men they may be of an erotic or ambitious nature, but whenever it is possible to analyze the ambitious reveries they, too, may be found to belong to the erotic. All great actions and accomplishments, heroic or commercial, are generally done for the purpose of pleasing some woman and to be preferred to other men. That our patient is no exception to the rule is quite natural.

RECAPITULATION

We have here a man of thirty-nine years old suffering from a psychosis of a year's duration. He cannot account for it. He thinks it came on suddenly. Only a few days before the onset he was thoughtful and nervous. This psychosis is characterized by two distinct crises with a transitional period of about five months. Both crises were of the delirious, confusional, dream-like type, the first lasting three days, and the second about one week. The period of transition is characterized by marked restlessness, delusions and hallucinations. The second crisis was not followed by any recovery in the strict sense, as he still entertained false ideas which he did not try to correct. On the contrary he considered all attempts in that direction futile and unnecessary. The strange manifestations he recognized as supernatural, divine and purposeful; they were intentionally sent to compel him to change his mode of living and return to the religion of his father. He sees in all this the "Hand of God." In other words, we see here a gradual and systematic change of personality which we have every reason to believe is only the process of transformation and will probably lead to further systematization and dissociation.*

Both the abstract of the history and the patient's katamnestic account give a fair gross picture of the psychosis, but do not in any way explain the psychogenesis of the symptoms. The associations, as can be seen, have thrown considerable light on the subject, they uncovered many obscure points and called forth many new ones, but we are still in darkness concerning the causal determinations of the symptoms which we shall now proceed to examine.

That the psychosis did not come on as suddenly as would appear is quite certain. When we thoroughly examine the patient's antecedent history we find that for a number of years his mind was gradually being prepared for it. Since his twenty-second year he sustained a number of psychic shocks of different degrees. The first and most important was his love affair with Miss B. which ended so unfortunately. To form an opinion of the effect it left on the patient it was only necessary to watch his mimic while he recited this episode. As we know it is very difficult to evoke an adequate affect in such patients, but when this unhappy love affair of sixteen years ago was touched he immediately lost his wonted taciturnity and indifference, his eyes brightened and his face reddened. He was again the young lover of twenty-two. He spoke fluently about his ardent affections: "I was then innocent and really loved. It was my first and true

* Nothing has been heard from the patient since his discharge from the hospital.

love. All the other love affairs which I subsequently entertained were dulled by this first one." He became enraged when he recalled his father's attitude in this affair. "Whenever I think of it I am compelled to hate him," he said. It is not difficult to see that this love was always in his mind in a repressed state and that it markedly influenced his actions.

In 1901 he loved another woman, Miss I. W. "It was only sexual love," he said, "but I would have married her." She proved false to him and married an army officer. In 1903 he decided to marry his landlady and his father again objected. This time, however, he disregarded his father and resolved to follow his own inclinations. As a result his father severed all relations with him and he neither saw nor heard from him for three years, yet this did not seem to disturb him. Yet in spite of all he did not marry Mrs. W. For reasons unexplained he kept on putting it off until Christmas, 1907, when he finally resolved to save his money and marry her. But at the same time there was a reawakening of paternal sentiment. He sent his father letters and his photograph, but they were all returned. This irritated him and he decided never to write to him again. As we have shown he did not keep his resolutions.

Besides the episodes mentioned there were probably other psychical disturbances, but unfortunately the patient was not very communicative. We also see quite plainly that for a number of years he was subjected to a mental conflict. As a youth he was brought up amid religious surroundings: His father was antisemitic and naturally the same ideas were inculcated in the son.

When he became older he changed completely. He became an atheist and worked among Jews for eighteen years. He no longer attended church, but studied Nietzsche, Stirner and others. Now and then his father upbraided him for it, but without avail. That he did not entirely rid himself of his early religious training, but only repressed it, is shown by the fact that he kept on subscribing to an antisemitic journal and during the Dreyfus affair, he was the only anti-Dreyfussard in his office. He could not be convinced that Dreyfus was not guilty (symbolic actions). Unconsciously his early training remained in a dormant state. It is not at all easy for one who has been brought up in a certain religious atmosphere to his sixteenth year to entirely free himself from it. Many persons imagine that they are entirely emancipated from their early religious training and are manifestly so until a grave moment intervenes. Then, provided they are mentally strong, the repressed ideas reassert themselves. This accounts for the many so-called conversions and recantations during grave diseases or on death beds.

Both the patient's crises show some connection with religious events. Christmas, 1907, marks the manifest beginning of his restlessness. At this time his feelings toward his father suddenly changed. The suggestive dream referred to under Ass. 7 was on the evening of Good Friday and marked the beginning of the second attack.* The day following the dream he set out on the journey which finally landed him in the hospital of K.

We see, then, that we have at least two psychic instances

* The episode in Wagner's Parsifal is also centered around Good Friday.

of great moment which have long been repressed and which now suddenly reasserted themselves. The question arises—how did this come about? A personal predisposition is presupposed. The conflict existing for years caused an "abaisment du niveau mental" (Janet).[4] The repressed unconscious complexes gradually freed themselves from the domination of the ego-complex[5] and then manifested themselves in the form of automatisms, such as suggestions and inspirations and finally as hallucinations. The obnubilation which followed allowed the appearance of the manifold senseless manifestations which were brought about by the dream mechanisms of Freud.

If this supposition is true, the individual symptoms ought to be psychically constellated by the complexes. I shall forthwith show that this is really the case.

When we look at our cases in the wards we are often struck by their strange utterances and peculiar behaviour. Until recently we were quite satisfied to note that the patient is delusional and demented, that he utters senseless phrases and goes through a number of peculiar actions. Thanks to Freud we know that all actions and speech in both normal and abnormal individuals are psychically determined.[6] Jung, following Freud, made thorough analyses of cases of Dementia Præcox showing that all the patients' absurd utterings were quite relevant when analyzed and, furthermore, that all the speech and motor manifestations were distinctly traced to the complex.[7]

Let us now examine the individual symptoms of our patient. The crises which we went through can be readily compared to the normal dream. Like the expressions in dreams our patient's utterances at first sight seem quite senseless, but have a meaning as soon as analyzed. The first crisis began with an ecstatic feeling. He was forced into an attitude of prayer by an invisible force. He had to cry out, "Lord, have mercy on suffering humanity." This is nothing but a powerful reassertion of his repressed religious presentations, which by his impaired judgment can only be interpreted as an external power. The complex of religion gained the upper hand and he was therefore forced to assume an attitude of prayer and cry out, "Lord, have mercy, etc." He also had to repeat the "Our Father" hundreds of times. As we know his father played a great part in this attack, hence the frequent repetition. The directing thought being absent the vacuum of association causes the stereotyped repetition. It must also be remembered that he identified himself with Christ and his father with God. Hence he repeated the Lord's prayer.

The influence of the Egyptian gods, Isis and Osiris, is explained in Ass. 53. The death of Mr. Osiris naturally interested him as he was a bank official. It is quite likely that either consciously or unconsciously he expressed a wish that some of the money would be left to him. The delirium, like the dream, fulfilled that wish and he, therefore, imagined that the banker left him thirty million francs. Osiris, is a contiguous association of Isis. Hence he felt the influence of Isis and Osiris.

Why was he forced to repeat "Am I Parsifal, the guileless fool?" In order to understand this analysis it is necessary to bear in mind the original German. He kept on repeating "Am I Parsifal reinster Thor." Those acquainted with Freud's methods of analyzing dreams know what a great part is played by "condensation" and "contamination."* On carefully examining the patient's doings of the day before his first crisis it was found that on looking over some old papers and correspondence he found many letters from his old sweetheart. He stated that he did not attempt to read them, but he happened to notice the following sentence: "I am in Pittsburgh, Pennsylvania, with a family named Thaw." This was the first letter she sent him from America in which she told him that she was a servant in the Thaw family. She remained with this family for some time and he corresponded with her regularly for about a year. He stated that after noticing this sentence it "sort of possessed him" and for hours he was compelled to repeat in his mind "Pittsburgh, Pennsylvania, Thaw." He spoke English fairly well and had a very good reading knowledge of it. On being requested to write this phrase he wrote it as follows: "Pa., Pittsburgh, Thaw," remarking at the same time that Pa. is the abbreviation for Pennsylvania. I now venture the following explanation. The memory picture of the word Pennsylvania may be the whole word or its abbreviation Pa., hence in the mind they exist simultaneously as Pa., Pennsylvania. The dream does not find it difficult to condense Pa. Pennsylvania into Pannsylvania and then form it into PANNSYVLania which corresponds to Parsifal. The resemblance between Thaw and Thor is quite obvious. If we now place the two sentences parallel to each other we have the following:

* Condensation is a fusion of events, pictures, and elements of speech. Contamination is a fusion of speech only (Jung).

PANNSYVLania	Pittsburg	THAW
PARSIFAL	reinster	THOR

All letters for the pronunciation of "reinster" can readily be found in the word Pittsburgh and the remnant of Pennsylvania. Such condensations and transpositions happen quite frequently in dreams, especially if there be another determining factor. Our patient imperfectly identified himself with Parsifal as shown in Ass. 55.

"The Jews played some part in it" is all we could get from our patient. He insisted that he never had any differences with Jews. What part they played in his attack cannot be explained, but it may simply have been a forcible reassertion of his father's doctrines.

Thus we see that all the known senseless utterances of the first crisis are fairly well determined. Let us now turn to the second crisis.

He was quite sure that during the first attack he heard no distinct voices. Everything was accomplished by some strange power which he designates as magnetic electric mental suggestion. These suggestions, although abating after the first crisis, did not entirely cease. He said that he was all the time more or less under suggestions. On July 16 he reached K. and passed a very restless night there. He slept but little and was constantly troubled by frightful dreams.

Only since Freud gave out his very profound and excellent work "The Interpretation of Dreams" can dreams be scientifically interpreted and those proficient in his methods possess an invaluable instrument for the exploration of the mind. When the patient was asked to recount the dreams he only remembered about "climbing a high mountain or mountains," that he suddenly became "like nailed" and could go no further and that he "experienced intense fear." (On another occasion be claimed to have dreamed about round arms and breasts. See explanation of Ass. 43.) When an attempt was made to analyze it he absolutely refused all collaboration. Notwithstanding this we know enough about dreams to enable us to venture an opinion. Since the first crisis he was under great mental stress. The conflict was "Shall I abide by my decisions and marry Mrs. W. or shall I comply with my father's wishes." As we know he had for years planned to marry in spite of his father's objections and about Christmas time was fully determined to do it when a sudden reaction set in and his repressed complexes predominated. The mountain climbing is a symbolic representation of this struggle. He was about to consummate his determination when he became "like nailed and could go no further." In the dream the sensation of being inhibited, such as not being able to move or run when one most desires to do so, means "no." There is a conflict of the will. One begins to do something and the censor says "No, that shall not be done." He was about to overcome all parental scruples. After years he finally decided to disregard his father and marry when he was suddenly checked.

This is quite a plausible and innocent interpretation, but like every harmless self evident dream it is only concealing something deeper and more intimate. The fear and anxiety in this dream show us that we deal with intense psychic resistance the content of which belongs to the erotic. Dreams accompanied by fear always belong to the sexual. "Anxiety is a libidinous impulse emanating from the unconscious and inhibited by the fore-conscious." (Freud.) In the waking state we find its counterpart in the psychoneuroses.[8] We know also that he dreamed of "round arms and breasts." Round arms and breasts are woman's arms and breasts. The mountains or mountain in the dream probably meant "mons veneris." The German expression for mons veneris is well known to the patient. As shown above he also dreamed of Venus and of her birth. This shows the sexual part of the dream. This is further strengthened by the fact that since his first crisis he was a sexual abstainer. Suppressed sexuality manifests itself in fear.

The onset of the second crisis was even more intense than the first. It began with suggestions and soon merged into distinct voices. While dressing the suggestive thought "almost like a voice said 'jump from the fourth floor window and if you believe you will rise unharmed.'" Then another suggestion said "How can you do it—you are only a sinner." Here we see very nicely the marked activity of the unconscious and the part played by the teleological suggestions. Both Bleuler[9] and Jung[10] give nice examples of this mechanism. It is a quite common contrast automatism and generally manifests itself in strong dissociations. Here we see it at the height of the disease.

As soon as he left the hotel the suggestion changed into auditory hallucinations. It was impossible to find out the contents of the hallucinations, but during the analysis of Ass. 12 he stated that the voice said "water, drink water." This likely refers to the Atlantic (Ass. 7) or to his complex of drinking (see Ass. 2). We know, however, that the voices so terrified him as to cause him to apply for police protection.

What followed he remembers but dimly. He was in a delirious dreamlike state for about a week. He was in heaven. He heard indistinct voices and saw "many bluish angels." His father was God and he was Christ and his former Superintendent R., for whom he had no particular love, was the Holy Ghost. He was now reconciled to his father and his religion. This was a hyperbolic realization of the normal dream. Says Freud: "The conscious wish becomes a dream incitor only when it succeeds in arousing a similar unconscious one," and "The wish as represented in the dream must be an infantile one."[10] The wish realization in our patient's delirium certainly fulfils all these conditions. It sounds like a fragment of a child's conception of heaven and recalls such religious paintings as Hofmann's Ascension or Zuccaro's Christ Surrounded by Angels.

Thus the problems are solved. The repressed complexes now dominate the ego-complex and influence all thoughts and actions. His personality underwent a complete transformation. He was no longer a follower of Stirner but considered the "Ego and his Own" as dangerous. From the avowed philosopher and atheist he changed into the devout believer of the supernatural and hence his preferred quotation "There are more things in heaven and earth, doctor, than are dreamt of in your psychiatry."

Case. II.—A. St., twenty years old, law student and journalist, was admitted to my service in the clinic of psychiatry, Zurich, on

January 22, 1908. His friend and colleague stated that the patient was a Hungarian journalist who came to Zurich to study law. He was considered very diligent and brilliant, but somewhat eccentric. He seemed to have been depressed for some time, remaining in bed for days and taking very little nourishment, but for the previous two days he had shown some improvement. He attempted to shoot himself at about 12 o'clock on the day of admission. He discharged five shots and beyond grazing his shirt, striking a candle which stood near his bed and a picture of Ibsen on the opposite wall he did no damage. The reason for the attempted suicide was supposed to be unrequited love. In the beginning of December he had made the acquaintance of a lady student with whom he soon became infatuated. His love was not reciprocated so that he became despondent, neglected his work and uttered pessimistic and gloomy ideas. The informant stated that as soon as the shots were heard he ran into the room and found the patient lying on the bed in a delirious condition. He was confused, murmured to himself and asked meaningless questions, repeating "Where are the white horses?" The last question he also repeatedly put to the physician who was called in soon after the shooting.

An anamnesis was also obtained from the patient's father about a week later. He denied any psychic abnormalities in the family, but he himself was neuropathic and it was afterward learned that one of his daughters was hysterical. He stated that the patient was always somewhat delicate, but developed normally. As he grew up he was "indifferent, cold, seclusive and obdurate, but very bright." He was always at the head of his class. His teachers referred to him as a prodigy and his professors predicted a great future for him. At a very early age he manifested a great talent for writing and since his fifteenth year he had supported himself by journalism. His feuilletons were sought for by the leading Hungarian journals. Due to the divorce of his parents he had lived apart from them since his fifteenth year. He, however, kept on corresponding regularly with his father and paid him an occasional visit.

On admission the patient was exceedingly apathetic and took absolutely no interest in his surroundings. When addressed he showed some confusion. He seemed to be unable to comprehend the questions and his answers were monosyllabic and laconic. He did not care what would happen. "Do what you please," he would say.

In appearance he was under-developed and small. His head seemed too big for his body, probably due to his long, black hair which hung over his shoulders. The physical examination revealed nothing in particular. In the ward he was quiet and indifferent. He lay on his back motionless, either keeping his eyes shut or staring vacantly into space. He expressed no desires and when an attempt was made to draw him into conversation he became mute. He took very little nourishment and this only after much urging. When seen the next morning he was essentially unchanged. The nurse reported that he slept well, but paid absolutely no attention to anything.

The main features were dulness, apathy, somnolence and probably hallucinations as shown by his asking for white horses. This condition continued for four days after which he gradually became brighter and at the end of a few days more he was apparently his former self.

He was discharged on January 31 to go to Vienna with his father. Diagnosis, schizophrenia.*

We have here a precocious youth, slightly burdened by heredity, who, having been disappointed in love, lost his mental equilibrium and merged into schizophrenia. He made an unsuccessful attempt at suicide and later he was delirious and hallucinatory, uttering senseless stereotyped phrases. This was followed by a short period of apathy, mutism and dulness, after which he gradually improved.

As soon as conditions were favorable an attempt was made to draw the patient into conversation so as to have him explain some of the obscure points, but, as is generally the case, nothing of importance could be elicited. He was suspicious or simply unwilling to enter deeply into the questions. A hundred associations were therefore taken and analyzed by the psychanalytic method, *i.e.*, after the complexes were found I resorted to the contin-

* The patient has been perfectly well since his discharge from the hospital.

uous associations. The words employed were the usual 100 words used for psychanalytic and diagnostic purposes. Some of the words, however, were changed and others bearing directly on the incident were inserted.

The following are some of the associations obtained from the patient:

Stimulus Word	*Reaction*	*Time*	*Reproduction*
4. To suppose	Freedom	3.8	X
5. Pain	Bad	2.2	X
6. Lazy	Early	1.8	X
7. Moon	Sun	2.6	X
12. To frighten	Epilepsy	3.4	X
14. Tired	Rest	2.0	X
15. Intention	Evil	2.8	X
16. To dance	Polish	3.0	X
17. Eye	Eye	3.8	X
19. To aim	I	3.8	Candle

Ass. 4, "to suppose—freedom" refers to his complex of confinement. He supposes that he will soon be discharged from the hospital. Ass. 5, "pain—bad" explains that he had much pain over this love affair, but, as shown by the reaction time, it provoked no emotion whatever. Ass. 6, "lazy—early" refers to his being lazy. He never likes to rise mornings. It also recalls that he was too lazy to commit suicide in the morning and waited until noon. Ass. 7, "moon—sun" was explained as follows: While walking one day with Mina (his beloved), they stopped to look at a photograph representing a man and woman riding on a crescent (moon). At that time the position of the two young persons on the crescent rather pleased him, and he remarked to her that he would like to ride with her on the moon. He then recalled some things which he did not wish to explain—probably some erotic thoughts. Ass. 12, "to frighten—epilepsy" referred to an incident in the ward. An epileptic had a fit which frightened him as it was the first time he ever saw such thing. Ass. 14, "tired—rest" referred to his state before admission to the hospital. Ass. 16, "to dance—Polish" was explained as follows: "On Saturday evening, December 7, I went to the Polish dance where I met my three lady acquaintances, Heda, Mina and Dina. My main object in going there was to gather some material for an article on the life of the Russian and Polish students in Zurich." He stated that when he got there he saw Miss Dina, whom he had known for some time, in the company of some gentlemen. He was not indifferent to her. He always found "something pleasant in her." She impressed him differently from the others because she was somewhat outspoken. On a number of occasions she did not hesitate to tell him that he was only a poseur, etc., a thing which rather wounded his vanity. Yet, he did not know why, she continued to be of more interest to him than the others. For some reason when he noticed her at the dance he purposely turned to another direction, but did not lose sight of her. On that evening he felt some change coming over him. Of a usually cynical and taciturn disposition he suddenly became very cheerful and loquacious. The music exerted an unusual influence on him. He said and did things which are still enigmatical to him. The women especially pleased him and, realizing this, the words of Mephistopheles recurred to him: "Du siehst mit diesem Trank im Leibe, Bald Helenen in jedem Weibe." Many women seemed to make advances to him.

They sent him all kinds of notes and made flattering remarks about him. One elderly woman made such remarks as "Just see this handsome boy," etc. Another woman, totally unknown to him, sent him a senseless note about "loving, human and erring." Another sent him a gillyflower. On later losing his necktie he stuck this flower into his collar and wore it for the remainder of the evening. Another peculiar action was this: Everybody was requested to wear numbers which were distributed to everyone present. The gentleman and lady drawing the same numbers were supposed to exchange souvenir cards. When he received his number he scratched it out and wrote on the card a big "I" and this he wore the entire evening. He further recalled that he was very restless for a few days previous. He spent money uselessly, went to many concerts, felt freer than usual, and thought of traveling. Ass. 17 "eye—eye" refers to his own eye. He thought that his left eye was somewhat smaller than his right and this he considered a sign of paresis. This gave rise to a number of hypochondriacal and depressive ideas. In a letter written to his father long before this suicide episode took place he signed himself "Candidate for Paresis." Ass. 19, "to aim—I—candle" he explained as follows: "At the moment that I grasped the revolver I felt some fear, but aimed at my breast. The discharge confounded me. I was convinced that I had struck myself and dropped the revolver, but I immediately grasped it again and fired four times. I seemed to look for something to aim at. I remember distinctly aiming at the candle standing not far from the window and at a picture of a bust of Ibsen on the opposite wall." More of this later.

Stimulus Word	*Reaction*	*Time*	*Reproduction*
22. Modest	Violet	3.2	X
23. Ground	Seed	4.6	Onanism
27. Death	Accidentally	3.0	X
30. Bad	Very	3.2	Night
34. Pretty	Fairly	2.0	X
40. To crack	Arms	2.0	X
47. Weapon	Unskilled	3.6	X
48. Forget	Love	3.0	X
51. To dare	To win	3.8	X

Ass. 22, "modest—violet" was explained as follows: "The violet is a symbol of modesty. Miss Dina always repeated that I was not modest. Many people reproached me for the same thing, but I always sought refuge in Goethe who says 'only scamps are modest.'" Ass 23, "ground—seed—onanism." By way of explanation he quoted the Bible "He (Onan) spilled it on the ground lest that he should give seed." When asked whether he masturbated he at first denied it, but when told that the associations gave distinct evidence of it, he said: "Well, since you know it, I may as well tell you. I began to masturbate when I was fourteen and continued it up to about a year ago. I then knew what harm it did me and I stopped it." When asked in what way it affected him he said that he read or was told that one is liable to get paresis and many other diseases from it. Ass. 27, "death—accidentally" referred to his attempted suicide. He fitly remarked "I could have died through accident." Ass. 30, "bad—very—night" referred to the night of January 15, which he claimed to have passed very restlessly. He was frequently terrified by his rocking chair, the coverings on which made him think of the dying Bajazzo. On the 12th, Mina and the others went to see Bajazzo. He was to have gone, but at the last moment he changed his mind and remained at home. This also recalled a conversation with Dina. She told him that his mania for originality, etc., was simply a desire to pose. He retorted by saying: "but don't you think that there is something tragic even in the poser, in the comedy-playing Bajazzos. If they really perceive the real feeling, such apparent comedies may sometimes lead to tragedies." Ass. 34, "pretty—fairly" referred to Mina. Ass. 40, "to crack—arms" means the revolver with which he attempted suicide. This recalled his friend, R., concerning whom he had read that he had attempted suicide by shooting himself in the head. This happened some time before the Polish dance, and on the day of the dance he received a letter from his friend describing the attempted suicide and stating that it had concerned a woman, and that he was well. Ass. 47, "weapon—unskilled" refers to himself. He said "I never in my life used any firearms and when I made up my mind to kill myself I selected a pretty little revolver." Ass. 48, "forget—love." He said: "I am trying to forget my love." Ass. 51, "to dare—to win" was not explained. He began to speak about courage and daring and he suddenly stopped, not wishing to continue.

Stimulus Word	*Reaction*	*Time*	*Reproduction*
54. Quick	To press	2.4	X
55. Child	Big	3.2	X
56. Enjoy	Life	2.2	X
61. Stone	To cast	2.2	X

Stimulus Word	*Reaction*	*Time*	*Reproduction*
80. To understand	Saying	3.6	X
83. Sofa	To sit	2.8	Girls
87. Snake	Eve	3.4	X
94. To write	Feuilleton	3.2	Spirit
95. Horse	Ghost	3.0	Rosmersholm

Ass. 54, "quick—to press" referred to his suicide. He was frightened when he grasped the revolver so that he quickly pulled the trigger. Ass. 55, "child—big." Mina often called him a child, which greatly offended him as he considered himself a man "in every sense of the word." Ass. 56, "enjoy—life." He said "I was tired of living and wanted to die, but now I would like to be discharged so as to enjoy life. Ass. 61, "stone—to cast" recalled the sentence: "He that is without sin among you, let him cast the first stone." He always condemned persons who committed suicide. He never liked a play or a book where the heroes ended their lives. He thought of writing a different ending to Ibsen's Rosmersholm. Ass. 80, "to understand—saying"—the saying is, '"To understand all is to forgive all'—that is what she said to me when she rejected my proposal. Her friend told me afterward that she was abnormal and was unable to love any man." Ass. 83, "sofa—to sit—girls" referred to a dream which he had while in the hospital in which the three girls were sitting on a sofa, etc. Ass. 87, "snake—Eve." "A snake was the cause of Eve's fall," he said. "A cat and a snake are symbols of falsehood." Snake made him think of penis. Ass. 94, "to write—feuilleton—spirit" he explained thus: "When I decided to commit suicide I immediately thought of writing a number of articles, one a dialogue, a witty interview between A. St., the collaborator of the Pesti Naplo and his spirit. I also intended to write to Dina that just at Tshepurnoy (the reference is to Gorky's 'Children of the Sun') saved the honor of the veterinary surgeons by committing suicide, I saved the honor of the 'posers.'" Ass. 95, "horse—ghost—Rosmersholm" referred to the white horses which play such a part in Ibsen's Rosmersholm.

A brief examination of these associations shows that most of them belong to the erotic complexes. We are also struck by the slight emotivity manifested in the associations directly concerned with the love episode. This is especially striking when all the 100 associations are examined. Indeed, whereas the associations evoked very interesting and valuable points they gave us very little information about the principal episode, the supposed cause of this whole drama. The widest emotional excursions were connected with the complexes extraneous to this episode. From the twenty-nine associations given, twelve (7, 16, 19, 27, 34, 40, 47, 48, 54, 56, 80 and 83) bear directly on the drama, and on examination we find that the arithmetical average of the reaction time is 2.8 seconds, a very minimal increase over the normal, and, furthermore, there is only one failure of reproduction and that in association 19. This last, however, does not *sensu stricto*, belong to the episode, as we shall see later, so that this reduces still more the average. Translating this into association language we say that the so-called complex-indicators are entirely absent where you would most expect them. Indeed, when I reviewed the 100 associations originally taken I found that the twenty-nine selected are the only associations that in any way concern the case, the other seventy-one belonging to entirely different complexes. This simply indicates that there are, perhaps, other more forceful factors than the mere love affair, that some invisible psychic undercurrent may play a greater part than the supposed cause—love.

If we orient ourselves on the incidents appertaining to this love affair we find that long before the patient became infatuated with Mina he was acquainted with Dina. In his katamnestic account the patient says: "I was attracted to her—Dina—by more than mere sympathy. She was outspoken and called me a poseur, but I always liked to be in her company." Some time after he met Mina and Heda, who did not make any particular impression on him and it was not until the Polish dance that he really became acquainted with them. The first part of the evening he had no predilection, but as the night advanced Mina attracted him more than her friend. On going home the next morning he walked with Mina and he still was in the "Hellenic state," very cheerful and frolicsome, but nothing was said of love. There were, however, some allusions to "waltzing through life together," but that was said jocosely and in company. The "Hellenic state" he described as follows: "It seemed to me that I had no ponderance. I felt infinitely light, ethereal and contrary to my wonted cynicism. I then was infinitely good, well wishing to everything and everybody. I felt neither desire nor wishes. It was a drop of the blessed sea of eternal contentment." This apathetic euphoria continued until Sunday afternoon when he again met the ladies in the company of a gentleman. For some reason he immediately took a dislike to this man and his euphoria disappeared.

On returning to his room he felt "confused and could not account for my actions of last night and today." He tried to repose for a few hours, as he had an appointment with his friend to take the girls to the theater in the evening, but he was exceedingly restless and unable to remain in the room. That evening he went to the theater, but did not enjoy himself at all. The following days continued uneventful. He frequently saw Mina and her friend in the boarding house, but had no serious thoughts. On the contrary he recalled that on one occasion the thought of love came to him and he immediately suppressed it, saying to himself "Do not delude yourself. Be careful lest you lose your liberty. It would be like committing suicide." It was not until a few days before she was to leave Zurich for her Christmas vacation that he was cognizant of the fact that he was in love. He, however, doubted it. She left on the 20th and it was then that it became clear to him that he loved her. He was distracted, indifferent to everything and suddenly conceived the idea of taking to his bed. Before doing so he wrote her a letter in which he told her all and asked for a categoric answer. He remained in bed for three days in succession, during which time he ate but little and slept less. He was sure that she would reject his proposal, wept much and was obsessed by anxious thoughts. He then got up and immediately visited Dina. She again accused him of being a poseur and he said, "I am really a thorough poseur, I can delude even myself. I could commit most terrible acts, such as marrying or committing suicide." Following this visit he felt better. Mina's answer was rather equivocal. She "did not know what to say," etc. She returned on January 4, and "strange to say, when I saw her not only was I not surprised, but I even seemed to be indifferent." He continued to see her regularly, but they never broached the subject. From the 10th he was very excited and had some fever and spent most of the time in bed. "On the 14th Mina visited me and during our conversation she told me that she did not think she could be capable of loving any one. She left me at 11 p.m. The rest of the night I slept fairly well, but dreamed of Dina."

The following days he was very depressed and restless, took no interest in anything, ate and slept very little. On the 17th, while walking about aimlessly, he suddenly decided to commit suicide and at the same time he was speculating on the interesting and original letters that he would write before shooting himself. He did not know what he would write to Mina, but thought of writing to Dina, and also a dialogue, an interview between himself and his spirit. He decided to buy a revolver. "The money that I expected did not come," said he. "I then went to see Dina. I wanted to hear her repeat that I was nothing but a poseur, but she was not at home." A few hours later he again tried to visit her, but she was not at home. The following day—the 18th—he again called on her and again missed her. Sunday he passed restlessly, but was watched by a colleague who suspected him. On Monday, just about noon time he made the attempt. He waited until he saw Mina and Heda go into the dining room and then ran into his room, undressed, and went to bed. He did not lock the door and then attempted suicide as described above.

Analysis.—Strange as it may seem the psychanalysis shows that the love affair played a very little, if any part, in this whole syndrome. No matter how a person may try to conceal things he cannot hide his emotions and unconscious actions. The associations, like dreams, never lie. The complex indicators never fail to show the complex, that is, the emotionally accentuated presentations which are usually split off from consciousness and repressed in the unconscious. On superficial examination it may seem that the psychosis was caused by the love affair, but as soon as we enter more deeply into the question we are struck with the marked disproportion between the exciting cause and the reaction and we ask ourselves why should an insignificant love episode produce a psychosis in a young man who has made his way in the world since his fifteenth year as a student and journalist and who, from his own account, has had similar experiences before this? To be sure there are those who maintain that just this incongruity between noopsyche and thymopsyche is characteristic of dementia præcox, but one of the greatest achievements of psychanalysis is the fact that it conclusively shows that in neither the psychoneuroses nor the psychoses proper is there such a thing as incongruity between noopsyche and thymopsyche. Wherever a thorough examination is possible it is always found that the reaction is quite adequate and that it simply appears incongruous to us because we cannot or do not enter into the patient's psyche. Moreover, when we examine our patient's past we find that long before this last experience he was depressed and listless, remaining in bed for days at a time and that he evinced many peculiar actions. All this distinctly shows that the love episode was only one of many contributing exciting factors.

On reviewing the 100 associations we find that they refer to four principal complexes, namely, love, vanity, death and masturbation. Of these thirty-five belong to the death complex, twenty to the complex of masturbation, twelve to the vanity complex, and twelve to the love episode. In other words, death and masturbation are of paramount importance while the love episode plays only a subordinate part.

The love complex we have already discussed, and of his vanity both he himself and his father stated that he was always very vain and of an independent nature. He stated "I am not of an emotional nature. My parents reproached me for being heartless, vain and cold, saying that my blood was as cold as that of an Englishman and that I was too independent." The wounding of his vanity was always associated with his suicide. In his katamnestic account he stated: "I was suddenly struck with the idea of committing suicide and I immediately tried to find Dina so as to evoke from her the oft-repeated statement that I was a 'thorough irremediable poseur.'" He was also chagrined by Mina because she called him "child." He insisted that he was a man in the fullest sense of the word.

Psychanalysis of the complexes of death showed that for some inexplicable reason the patient had for some time both consciously and unconsciously, occupied himself with the problem of death. When asked to associate freely to the word "death" he gave the following reactions: "When we dead awaken"—he recalled his friend the actor, who was supposed to have blown out his brains—

Rosmersholm. On further analysis we found that "when we dead awaken" refers to Ibsen's drama of that title He stated that for some time this play strongly appealed to him, but since reading Rosmersholm the latter had exerted a greater influence over him. He, however, did not like the last act, and thought seriously of rewriting the play, giving it another ending. He despised persons like Rosmer and Rebecca for committing suicide. "They are not people of this world," he said, "they belong to the morbid, fanatic and romantic nations." While in the hospital he wrote to the author: "Do I perhaps suffer from neurasthenia or am I in the first stage of paresis? If so I will see that it will not progress." In a letter which he sent to his father long before this love episode occurred he signed himself "Candidate for Paresis." Moreover, for the previous year or so he signed his feuilletons with the following pseudonyms "Schakal," "Sansdieu," "Enfant Terrible" and "Sansculotte." Those who are unfamiliar with Freud's "Psychopathology of Every Day Life"[11] may consider our patient's use of the pseudonyms as purely accidental, but we have it from Freud that nothing is adventitious or arbitrary. Just such trivialities show us the real unconscious activity. These pseudonyms are the equivalent for "I am a jackal, godless," etc. That is to say, they represent delusions of self-accusation.

All that clearly shows that long before the love episode the patient was hypochondriacal and restless. He entertained a number of delusions of a depressive, somatopsychic and self-accusatory nature. He made a number of unsuccessful attempts to stop masturbating, for he thought that it would produce paresis, and when he finally noticed a slight difference in the size of his eyes he became firmly convinced that he was a paretic. He also heard and read much about paresis and, as we have shown, he soon began to occupy himself with the problem of death. Therefore, anything referring to it interested him. It was while in that state of mind that he fell in love with Mina and for a brief period there was a reaction, the "Hellenic state." This, however, soon disappeared and long before he knew that his love would not be reciprocated he again became depressed. This love episode was simply the "last straw to break the camel's back." That is, the conflict probably existed for years until finally a compromise formation took place and the result was the suicidal episode.

The situation, in brief, was as follows: "I am suffering from an incurable disease—paresis—which I brought upon myself by masturbation and as I will become insane I had better commit suicide." Added to that there was the wounding of his vanity by both Dina and Mina. Against all this, however, there was the inherent desire to live. In the language of Jung, the long-existing conflict in a personal predisposition finally produced a splitting of consciousness, or Janet's abaissement du niveau mental, thus allowing the repressed complexes to rid themselves of the domination of the ego complex and manifest themselves in the different automatisms of the syndrom.[12]

Let us now examine the psychic constellations of the individual symptoms. In the first place, we may ask why the patient chose this method of suicide? This was directly suggested to him by the shooting episode in the life of his friend, the actor. He, himself, had never before handled any firearm and there was absolutely no reason why he should have deferred this affair as he did for the purpose of getting money to buy a revolver. He had numerous other means within his reach. He could at any time have resorted to hanging, drowning or poisoning, which would have been easier to accomplish. Still he selected a method which was entirely foreign to him. When he bought the revolver he had to ask the storekeeper for instructions as to its use. I have it from Dr. M. S. Gregory, who has devoted considerable time to the subject, that suicides invariably follow a definite procedure. Thus soldiers and others who are accustomed to firearms always select pistols or revolvers for suicidal purposes; physicians, druggists and chemists invariably use poison, while ordinary persons follow some method suggested by suicidal incidents read in the daily press or they imitate some relative or friend. The same day that he attended the Polish dance he received a letter from his friend, telling him that he was alive and well, though he had attempted to blow out his brains on account of a woman.

According to Freud all delusional formations and actions are the result of a compromise. There are two psychic streams opposing each other and finally each yields a part of its demand and a mutual accommodation results. Our patient's suicidal attempt was simply symbolic. He really did not wish to terminate his life, though he wished to die. He simply wished to annihilate that part of himself which was most repugnant to him and which was responsible for his malady.

Association 19 shows that the patient aimed directly at the candle. On being asked to associate to candle he gave the following: "It recalls to me a picture of a big candle, a big white candle on a dark background. Candles always make me feel disagreeable. I used to avoid passing a certain store where there was a show case filled with candles. The burning candles with the dripping tallow which I used to see in churches and temples nauseated me. That recalled a girl named 'Baby S.' whom I used to know—that's all." When asked about this girl he showed numerous blockings and then continued: "She was anæmic and they used to say that—that she candled herself." Again blockings, but after considerable urging he stated that a candle with the dripping tallow recalls the penis after masturbation, a thing which always filled him with disgust. The resistance was broken and he frankly added: "That has been the bane of my life. I have not done it for a year because I was told that it would cause paresis."

The candle, as we see, is simply a symbolic representation of the penis. This is a familiar and widespread symbol, both in this country and abroad. The general popular belief that a virgin can relight with her breath a candle recently extinguished probably owes its origin to the same symbolic expression[13] (relight with her breath a candle—reawaken lost sexual powers).

Thus we see the reason for his aiming at the candle. In destroying the candle he killed that part of himself which is at the basis of all his trouble.

Why did he aim at Ibsen's picture? In order to understand this it is necessary to cite a fragment of a long dream which the patient had while in the hospital. It was as follows: "I got a harp and played something melancholic and the doctor stood there watching me and then exclaimed, 'Behold a lion's head arising on a feeble body,' and then wishing to hide his feelings he turned away." According to Freud, whenever one hears some speech in the dream it generally signifies that the dreamer has heard at some time the exact or similar words. The words which he puts in the doctor's mouth he actually heard from the doctor. On seeing the patient for the first time, while he was still in the somnolent state, I was struck by the size of his head and I remarked to the supervisor "He looks ill and is underdeveloped. His head seems too big for his body." In the dream this is changed to a lion's head. On analyzing the expression "lion's head" we obtained the following: "Head of a lion—Max Lieberman, a German painter, made a picture of a sphinx with the head of Ibsen on it—it looks like a lion's head—thinks of his own head which he believes "perhaps resembles Ibsen's head." On further analysis he identified himself directly with the great poet and stated that he noticed the resemblance between himself and Ibsen and that is why he bought the picture. We can now understand why he shot at the picture, for in doing so he again symbolically shot himself. We also know that for more than a year he took great interest in Ibsen's works, especially "When We Dead Awaken" and "Rosmersholm." This, too, as mentioned above, is a symbolic action. The title of the former play appealed to him because, believing that he was suffering from an incurable disease and that he would soon die, he naturally speculated on "When We Dead Awaken."

Such symbolic actions are frequently observed in everyday life. Only within a few days the daily press reported the case of a New York embezzler who was discovered by detectives in a Philadelphia public library. The book which he was reading at the time of his arrest was entitled "Will I Ever Go Back?" Rosmersholm, too, appealed to him because he directly identified himself with Rosmer "the happy nobleman who goes to death," but as the "will to live" always predominated in him he at first disliked the suicide of the lovers and even thought of rewriting the last act.

What was the origin of the stereotype "Where are the white horses?" Those who have read Ibsen's drama will recall that whenever a death occurred in Rosmersholm the white horse was sure to make its appearance. As our patient identified himself with Rosmer and lived through the tragic end of the "happy nobleman" he looked for the white horse in his delirium and hence the stereotyped question, "Where are the white horses?"

Thus we see that there was nothing mysterious or senseless in our patient's actions. All these actions and utterances had a reason and followed the same course as that of any normal individual. Indeed, those who make use of the psychanalytic method are well aware of the fact that whenever the patient's mind can be entered he ceases to be an enigma and his "senseless actions and utterances" cease to appear senseless. On the contrary we are often struck with the purposeful, nay ingenious, construction of the whole scheme. Moreover, we are always sure to miss —that "garbage can" of mental diseases—the "dementia" which is supposed to be the main characteristic of the disease. I have not seen a single analyzable case of dementia præcox that showed any dementia. Those cases whose minds we cannot penetrate merely because the patients refuse to cooperate with us we are hardly justified in calling "demented." Every careful observer will recall that now and then a "dement," who has been noted for years with the familiar formula "No change, dull, stupid, and demented," suddenly loses his dementia and acts in a perfectly rational manner. I can now recall three cases of dementia præcox that I observed in the Central Islip State Hospital which were "demented" two, three and five years, respectively, and then fully recovered, which led me to believe in the truth of the statement that dementia præcox is often "neither a dementia nor a præcox." The works of the Zurich school and of other investigators have amply demonstrated these facts and it is for these reasons that my former chief, Prof. Bleuler, to whom I am indebted for these cases, repudiates this meaningless term, dementia præcox, and uses Schizophrenia.[14]

References

1. Diagnostiche Assoziations Studien, Vol. I, Barth, Leipzig, 1906.

2. Translated by A. A. Brill, American Journal of Psychology, April, 1910.

3. Freud: Selected Papers on Hysteria, p. 194.

4. Janet: Les Obsessions et la Psychasthenie, Paris, 1903.

5. The Psychology of Dementia Præcox. Translated by Peterson and Brill.

6. Freud: *L. c.*, p. 165.

7. Jung: *L. c.*

8. *Cf.* Chap. III.

9. Bewusstsein u. Assoziation, Diagnost. Assoziations Studien, Beitrag V. and Jung, *L. c.*

10. The Interpretation of Dream, Translated by A. A. Brill, George Allen, London, and The Macmillan Co., New York.

11. *Cf.* Chap. VII.

12. Jung: *L. c.*

13. Liebman: Christlichen Symbolic, p. 76, Leipzig, Reklam Ed.

14. Bleuler: Schizophrenie, Deuticke, Wien, 1911.

CHAPTER VI

PSYCHOLOGICAL MECHANISMS OF PARANOIA

Its Relation to Homosexual Wish-phantasies

The subject of paranoia has always been a puzzle for psychiatrists and much has been said and written about it, but as far as my knowledge of the literature goes no real attempt or progress has been made toward its solution. For those who are acquainted with the subject no further dilatation is necessary. The others will have to be content with these statements, as it is not my purpose to enter here into an extensive discussion on the subject of paranoia in general.

Before entering into the psychological elements of the subject I will cite the following case:

E. R., thirty-six years old, married, school teacher by occupation, was admitted to my service at the Central Islip State Hospital, August 31, 1906. He came by transfer from the Bloomingdale Hospital where he had been for some time. In brief the history of the case taken from commitment papers was as follows: In infancy the patient sustained a severe fall on the head, but without apparent injury. In childhood he was subject to violent fits of temper. He would strike his head against the wall when angry and is supposed to have had some fainting attacks when frightened. At an early age he was employed in a factory. He resented his vulgar surroundings and blamed his relatives for permitting him to work there. He entered college at sixteen and worked his way through. He stood well in his classes, but was not popular with his classmates. He often quarreled with them and assumed a high moral plane. He refused to accompany them on frolics because he would not visit common places. He graduated in 1898 and then took up school teaching. Here, too, he did not seem to get along well with his principal and other teachers. He was disappointed at not being promoted to teach a higher grade and suspected that there was a conspiracy against him. He imagined that the principal and other teachers were trying to work up a "badger game" on him to the effect that he had had some immoral relations with his girl pupils. As a result of these delusions he would not permit his girl pupils to come near him in the school room. In 1903 he married, after a hasty courtship, and soon thereafter he took a strong dislike to his brother-in-law and sister and accused them of immorality. He also accused his wife of illicit relations with his brother and his brother-in-law, Mr. S. These erotic delusions, in conjunction with many other delusions of self-reference and persecution, became very active. The patient threatened to shoot his imaginary persecutors, so that it became necessary to commit him to Bloomingdale Hospital. There he remained from March, 1906, to June, 1906, when he was taken home on a trial visit, but as he soon began to react to his delusions and became excited and threatening, he was returned to the hospital after two days. One of his peculiar delusions at that time was that Dr. D., the physician in charge, was his wife in disguise.

When he was brought to the Central Islip State Hospital he was quite calm and natural in his conversation. As we had been classmates at college we were both pleased and sorry to meet under the circumstances. He spoke freely about his condition, but he denied, or tried to explain away his many delusions. Without entering into the details of his behavior during the four months he was under my care, I will merely state that he presented a typical case of paranoia. Mr. S., his brother-in-law, was the arch conspirator against him. He accused him of immoral relations with his wife and his mother and Mrs. S., *i.e.*, patient's sister. He often imagined that I was his wife in disguise and on a number of occasions he also accused his brother of being his wife in disguise. The following notes taken from the patient's history nicely illustrate that point: "On Sept. 6, 1906, while speaking to me, he said: 'Suppose I should tell you that my brother who visited me last Saturday and Doctor Brill were both Mrs. R. (wife) in disguise. . . . . . Doctor may I ask you a frank question?' When told to do so he said, 'Did you really have an interview with me last Sunday or is it only another case of Doctor Jekyl and Mr. Hyde? You don't look to-day as you looked then. You had all the feminine traits of Mrs. R.; to-day you are severe and look like yourself.'"

He also imagined that some women made signs to him and were in the hospital for the purpose of liberating him. Whenever he heard anybody talking he immediately referred it to himself. He interpreted every movement and expression as having some special meaning for himself. There was no impairment of his orientation or reasoning power. Contrary to the advice of the physicians he was discharged December 11, 1906.

It will hardly be worth while to enter into the further particulars of the symptomatology of this case. I will simply relate the following facts: In the summer of 1908 the patient was returned to Bellevue Hospital by his own family because he was very delusional and because they considered him dangerous. After having been there over three months and after a long trial before a jury in the Supreme court where five physicians, including myself, had testified that he was a dangerous paranoiac, he was declared sane and congratulated by the Supreme Court justice and the jury on his able management of his own case. He did not wait for his official discharge from the psychopathic ward of Bellevue Hospital, but escaped to Canada. His psychosis was apparently progressing for every now and then he would send mysterious letters to different persons in New York City. At that time one of his delusions was that he was a great statesman and that the United States government had appointed him ambassador, but that the "gang" in New York City had someone without ability to impersonate him so that he lost his appointment. This led him to send many letters to the State Department at Washington. On one occasion he appeared there and made an unsuccessful attempt to see the President's daughter. He was arrested by the secret service men and returned to New York, but again a judge allowed him to remain at large. He immediately returned to Canada and continued to annoy the Canadian government with all kinds of crazy letters. The Canadian government was quicker than a New York Supreme Court jury to recognize a lunatic, for he was arrested, declared insane and deported to the United States as an undesirable alien. He was again brought to the psychopathic ward in Bellevue where I had occasion to examine him. He expressed his former delusions, but they were more systematized and complicated. He showed considerable mental deterioration, so that he was unable to hide his delusions. He thought that the daughter of the President of the United States came to visit him in the hospital and he spoke quite freely about it. Indeed, the psychosis was so apparent that he was soon adjudged insane and committed to the Manhattan State Hospital.

The characteristic development, the delusions of persecution, the erotomania (girl pupils, President's daughter, and many women who came to set him free from the Central Islip State Hospital) and the delusions of grandeur (statesman, ambassador) present a typical picture of a paranoid condition.

I have not seen the patient for more than two years, but I am quite sure that very little new light has been thrown on the case since then. Now I do not expect to clear up all the obscure points in this case. All I hope to do is to demonstrate thereby certain mechanisms brought out by Freud in his psychanalytical remarks on a Case of Paranoia[1] and at the same time to give a rather full review of Freud's paper in order to stimulate further interest in this subject.

According to Freud the paranoiac character lies in the fact that as a reaction to a defense against a homosexual wish-phantasy there results a delusion of persecution. This conclusion has been reached not only by Freud, but also by Jung, Ferenczi,[2] and Maeder,[3] after having observed for years a number of cases of paranoia in men and women of different races, callings and social positions. This statement may seem strange on superficial consideration, as it is generally known that the etiological factors usually found in paranoia deal rather more with social injuries and depreciations than with matters sexual, but if we trace the social relations and at the same time bear in mind Freud's idea of sexuality we find that they invariably lead to unconscious homosexual wish-phantasies.

Studies made by Freud[4] and Sadger[5] have called attention to a stage in the history of the development of the libido which is passed on the way from autoerotism to object love. This stage has been designated as narcism and consists in the fact that the developing individual, while collecting into a unit his active autoerotic sexual impulses in order to gain a love object, takes first himself, his own body, as the object love, before going over to the object selection of a strange person. This intermediate phase between autoerotism and object love is normally perhaps indispensable, and in a great many persons it lasts for a long time. The genitals may then be the chief thing in this self which is taken as the love object. The remaining road may lead to the choice of an object with similar genitals and then from the homosexual object selection to the heterosexual. It is assumed that those who remained homosexual were unable to free themselves from the desire of requiring genitals similar to their own in the object love. This desire is also furthered by the infantile sexual theories which adjudge the penis to both sexes. In the normal course of development where the heterosexual object selection has been attained the homosexual feelings are not necessarily abrogated or suspended, but they are simply pushed away from the sexual aim and directed to new uses. They help in the formation of those components which constitute the social feelings and thus contribute to the maintenance of friendship, *camaraderie* and public spirit. This is the so-called process of sublimation. All the manifest homosexuals who resist their sensual feeling take an unusual interest in human affairs.

In his "Three Contributions to the Sexual Theory," Freud states that every stage of development of the psychosexuality offers a possibility for "fixation" which may thus result in a type of character. Persons who do not get away altogether from the stage of narcism, who are fixed there on some point which may act as a morbid disposition, are exposed to the danger lest a high tide of libido, finding no other outlet, might subject their social feelings to a sexualization and thus cause a retrogression of their sublimation which was acquired during the development. Such a state may come about by anything that produces a backward coursing of the libido (regression). It may be brought about by a collateral reinforcement through a disappointment in the woman, or through a failure in social relations to the man, or through a general increase in libido which becomes too violent to be discharged by the roads open to it and hence breaks the dam at the weakest portion of the structure. As analysis shows that paranoiacs endeavor to defend themselves against such a sexualization of their social feelings, the assumption forces itself that the weak part of their development is to be found in the parts between autoerotism, narcism and homosexuality. It is there that their morbid disposition lies. When we read the personal history of E. R. we find the following passages: "At an early age he was employed in a factory. He resented the vulgar surroundings and blamed his relatives for permitting him to work there. At sixteen years of age he decided to enter college and he worked his way through. He worked hard and stood well in the class. He quarreled with classmates and assumed a high moral plane. He would not visit common places when friends went on a frolic, etc."

In other words, there seems to have been some fixation at the phases of autoerotism and narcism, and a failure of sublimation of his homosexual component. I well remember how shut in and seclusive he was while at college. During the noon recess when the students would chat together in small groups he could be seen standing alone near some wall. As far as I know he did not have a single friend. From his history we gather that the psychosis became manifest as soon as he began teaching school, *i.e.*, as soon as an adjustment to environment was necessary. For adjustment to environments is nothing but a reaction to social stimuli. It is nothing but a give and take of libido. Here no transference was possible because his sublimation was made retrogressive and all his social feelings were sexualized. The reaction against his unconscious homosexual wish-phantasy caused him to think that he was slighted by his principal and the other teachers. In his own words—"they were trying to work up a badger game" on him. The normal relations between teacher and pupil became impossible. He would not permit his girl pupils to come near him because he thought they had some designs on him. This simply means that he previously entertained some sexual ideas about them or they probably represented a fixation from an early age.

In 1903 he married after a short courtship. He soon began to accuse his wife of infidelity with his brother and brother-in-law, Mr. S. He also accused Mr. S. of improper relations with his own wife (patient's sister) and a few years later he also accused him of improper relations with his mother. S. was the arch conspirator and his brother who was also one of the conspirators was under S.'s influence. There was apparently a conflict between his conscious heterosexuality and his unconscious homosexuality. For a time his heterosexuality triumphed and he married after a short courtship, but the unconscious homosexuality gained the upper hand and he then began to accuse his wife of infidelity with those men whom he himself unconsciously loved, *i.e.*, he projected his homosexuality to his wife.

But[6] when we accept the homosexual wish-phantasy to love the man as the nucleus of the conflict in paranoia of men, we at once find that it is contradicted by all the familiar principal forms of paranoia. Thus the sentence "I love him" (the man) is contradicted by the delusion of persecution which loudly proclaims "I do not love him —I rather hate him." However, the mechanism of the symptom formation in paranoia demands that the inner perception, the feeling, should be replaced by a perception from without. The sentence "I rather hate him" therefore becomes transformed through projection into the sentence "he hates (persecutes) me which justifies my hating him." The active unconscious feeling thus appears as a result of an outer perception "I really do not love him—I hate him—because he persecutes me."

Observation leaves no doubt that the persecutor was once loved and respected. One of my paranoid patients, D. S., talked about his arch conspirator Healy as follows: "I wanted him to take off all the influences, but he would not do it. . . . . . I had all sorts of pains around the heart and I thought I would die. I felt like dropping. I had lots of night losses. I was always drawn to him. I couldn't keep away from him." (Note the association between night losses and being drawn to him.)

Another point of attack for the contradiction is the erotomania which maintains "I do not love him—I love them." (E. R. always maintained that many ladies came to help him and that the president's daughter was in love with him, etc.). But the same impulsion to projection changes the sentence into "I notice that they love me." We then have "I do not love him—I love her—because she loves me." Many cases of erotomania could give the impression of exaggerated or distorted heterosexual fixation if we were not aware of the fact that all these loves do not start with inner perceptions of loving, but are feelings of being loved coming from without. Thus R., a stage hand who was committed to the Central Islip Hospital because he imagined that a certain well-known actress was in love with him and who annoyed her with his attentions, excused himself by saying that he was sure she loved him. Otherwise, he said, he would not have forced his attention on her. He was, however, unable to mention a single instance to justify his statement.

The third contradiction would be the delusions of jealousy which were also present in our patient.

In the delusions of jealousy of alcoholics we fully understand the part played by alcohol. It removes inhibitions and causes a regression of sublimation. *In vino veritas.* The man is often driven to drink through disappointment in the woman, which usually means he goes to the saloon or club in the company of men who give him the emotional gratification which he misses at home. But as soon as the men become objects of a stronger libidinous occupation in his unconscious he defends himself through a third form of contradiction "Not I love the man—she loves *him*," and he then suspects his wife with all the men he attempted to love. In our patient, who is a total abstainer, the alcohol naturally played no part.

One may now think that the three links of a sentence "I love him" would only admit three forms of contradiction, viz., the delusions of jealousy contradict the subject; the delusions of persecutions, the verb, and the erotomania, the object. However, there is still a fourth form of contradiction forming the total rejection of the whole sentence. The sentence reads: I do not love at all, and hence I love nobody, and as the libido must be somewhere the sentence is psychologically equivalent to the sentence: "I only love myself." This form of contradiction results in the delusion of grandeur which we conceive as a sexual overestimation of one's own ego and which can be put side by side with the familiar overestimation of the love object.[7] In our patient that manifests itself in his delusions of being an ambassador and many similar ones.

We can now understand some of the patient's delusions. Mr. S., his brother-in-law, was at first one of his best friends. The unconscious homosexual transference went too far and in his defense against it, the projection mechanism turns S. into a persecutor. What are the contents of the persecution? The patient answers this as follows: "He is trying to ruin my home and my own immediate family, that is my wife and sister . . . . . he is not a good man . . . . . I accuse him of improper relations with my sister (that is, his own wife). (Taken from hospital records.)

I could not elicit from the patient what these improper relations were. Whenever I broached the subject he became excited, but uncommunicative. On a number of occasions, however, he directly accused Mr. S. of being a pervert and a degenerate. That points to the fact that the improper relations were of that nature, for what other relations between husband and wife could be considered improper?

I here call your attention to a very important psychological mechanism, the mechanism of identification. Freuds tells us that the identification mechanism enables the patients to represent in their symptoms the experience of a great number of persons. They can suffer, as it were, for a whole mass of people and impersonate all the parts of a drama by means of their individual resources. It is not the simple hysterical imitation, but an unconscious mechanism. It is a sympathy based upon the same etological claims. It expresses an "as though" and refers to something common which has remained in the unconscious. In hysteria we know identification is most often used to express sexual community. Hysterics identify themselves most easily with persons with whom they had real or imaginary sexual relations or with those who had sexual relations with the same person.[8] Bearing in mind this mechanism we must conclude that the three persons suspected of sexual relations with S. must have some community to the patient. This, of course, is not difficult to divine. We all know that mother, sister, and wife are often identified even in the normal.[9] He was once in love with all of them, but as they could not gratify him, he unconsciously turned to homosexuality, to S. However, as he had suppressed the unconscious homosexual wish feeling for S., he then consciously perceived that not he loves S, but they love him. In other words, an inner perception was suppressed and as a substitute its content came to consciousness as an outer perception after it had been subjected to disfigurement. This is the mechanism of projection. This identification could also be found in his other delusions as the psychosis continued to progress. While in the Bloomingdale Hospital he imagined that Dr. D. was his wife in disguise. In the Central Islip Hospital he imagined that I was his wife in disguise. One incident in particular illustrates this point. On one occasion I made my night rounds at 11.30 o'clock, rather later than usual. He detained me for some time with many irrelevant questions. The next morning the supervisor brought me a letter which he wrote to his wife in which there was the following passage, "I am very sorry for having been so rude last night, but it was not my fault. Why did you appear disguised as Dr. Brill in a strange uniform? Why can't you come to me in your own sweet form?" Why did he think that the doctors were his wife in disguise? This question is very simple when we think of the mechanism of transference in reference to doctor and patient, with which I hope all my readers are familiar.[10] From my own experience with our patient I know that the transference first took the same course as in any neurosis, but as the patient defended himself against this homosexual wish-phantasy, he at first identified the doctor with his wife and then the idea was "I do not love him, but her. It is not Dr. D. or Dr. Brill. It is my wife." But as the psychosis progressed it was then transformed into the idea "I do not love him—I rather hate him because he persecutes me," which actually turned out to be the case. After the patient was recommitted to Bellevue Hospital he told me that I was one of the "gang." I was no longer his wife in disguise, but his enemy. The distortion that took place in the projection mechanism was an emotional transformation. What should have been perceived as love subjectively was perceived as hatred objectively.

But as the mechanism of projection does not play the same part in all forms of paranoia and as it is also found in other psychic occurrences such as in the normal we cannot consider it the most essential and pathognomonic element of paranoia. Let us therefore temporarily leave the study of projection and with it the mechanism of the paranoic symptom formation and turn our attention to the form of repression which is more intimately connected with the development of the libido and its contained disposition than with the form of the symptom formation.

A more thorough examination shows that the process of repression can be divided into three phases. The first phase consists in fixation which is the forerunner and the determination of every repression. The fact of fixation may be expressed by stating that an impulse or part thereof does not experience what may be regarded as normal development andconsequently remains in an infantile stage. Its libidinous emanation behaves toward the later psychic formations as if it belonged to the system of the unconscious, or as if it were repressed. Such fixation of the impulses may already contain the disposition for the later disease and above all the determinations for the failure of the third phase of the repression.

The second phase of the repression is the actual repression which we have hitherto had in mind. It emanates from the more highly developed conscious systems of the ego and may be designated as an "after repression." It gives the impression of a real active process, whereas the fixation is represented as a passive backwardness. Repression affects either the psychic descendants of those primary impulses which have remained backward if by virtue of their enforcement they come into conflict with the ego (or with its proper impulses) or with such psychic feelings against which there is a strong antipathy for other reasons. This aversion, however, would not result in repression if there should not already exist some connection between the repugnant strivings to be repressed and those already repressed.

The third phase is the failure of the repression, the breaking through, or the return of the repression. This breaking through results from the point of fixation and manifests a regression of the development of the libido up to this point. It stands to reason that there may be as many fixations as there are stages of development of the libido.

It is impossible to demonstrate these minute mechanisms in our patient. As I said above, I have not seen him for years, so that I am unable to tell what has taken place since then. In his profound analysis of the case of Schreber, Freud shows that even after the patient returned to society and found that he was mistaken in his idea that the world came to an end, he was nevertheless certain that the world had come to an end while he was sick and what he now saw before him was not really the same world. Such transformations of the world are quite common in paranoia. I know a number of paranoiacs who went through a stormy period lasting for years, but who now live contentedly, as if in another world. They do not care for anything, as nothing is real to them. They have withdrawn their sum of libido from the persons of their environment and the outer world. The end of the world is the projection of this internal catastrophe. Their subjective world came to an end since they withdrew their love from it. By a secondary rationalization the patients then explain whatever obtrudes itself upon them as something intangible and fit it in with their own system. Thus one of my paranoid patients who considers himself a sort of Messiah denies the reality of his own parents by saying that they are only shadows made by his enemy, the devil, whom he has not yet entirely subdued. Another paranoiac, in the Central Islip State Hospital, who represented himself a second Christ, spends most of his time sewing out on cloth crude scenes containing many buildings interspersed with pictures of the doctors. He explained all this very minutely as the new world system, and although he labeled the doctors with their proper names he nevertheless maintained that they were other persons concerning whom he knew much that could not be told. Thus the paranoiac builds up again with his delusions a new world in which he can live. The delusional formations which we take up as the morbid productions are, in reality, a curative attempt, a reconstruction as it were. The patient usually succeeds in accomplishing this after the catastrophe, and in this way he regains his relations to the persons and things of this world. Hence the process of repression consists in a withdrawal of the libido from persons and things that were previously loved. This is brought about mutely and without our knowledge. What we perceive as the disturbance is really the curative process, which makes the repression retrogressive and reconducts the libido to the persons it originally left. It is brought about in paranoia by way of projection. It was therefore incorrect to say that the inner suppressed feelings are outwardly projected. It is better to say that what was inwardly suspended returns from without.

However,[11] a withdrawal of libido is not an exclusive occurrence in paranoia, nor does its occurrence anywhere necessarily follow by disastrous consequences. Indeed, in normal life, there is a constant withdrawal of libido from persons and objects without resulting in paranoia or other neuroses. It merely causes a special psychic mood. The withdrawal of libido as such cannot therefore be considered as pathogenic of paranoia. It requires a special character to distinguish the paranoiac withdrawal of libido from other kinds of the same process. This is readily found when we follow the further utilization of the libido thus withdrawn. Normally we immediately seek a substitute for the suspended attachment and until one is found the libido floats freely in the psyche and causes tensions which influence our moods. In hysteria the freed sum of libido becomes transformed into bodily innervations or fear. Clinical indications teach us that in paranoia a special use is made of the libido which is withdrawn from the object. We know that most cases of paranoia evince delusions of grandeur and that the delusions of grandeur may themselves constitute a paranoia. From this we conclude that the freed libido in paranoia is thrown back on the ego and serves to magnify it. Thus it again reaches to the familiar stage of narcism from the development of the libido in which one's own ego was the only sexual object. "It is this clinical fact that teaches us that paranoiacs have brought along a *fixation in narcism* and we therefore assert that the *return from the sublimated homosexuality to narcism* furnishes the *sum of regression* which is characteristic for paranoia."[12]

The near relations between paranoia and dementia præcox are as follows: Paranoia is to be considered an independent clinical type notwithstanding the fact that it is complicated by schizophrenic features. Considered under the guise of the libido-theory it is distinguished from dementia præcox by another localization of the predisposed fixation and by another mechanism of the return (symptom formation). The principal character of the actual repression—the removal of the libido and regression to the ego—is common to both. Abraham has thoroughly demonstrated that the character of the withdrawal of the libido from the other world is especially clear. From this character we infer that the repression is brought about by the withdrawal of libido. The phase of active hallucinations is to be conceived as a struggle between the repression and the effort toward a cure which is to bring back the libido to its object. But this striving toward adjustment does not make use of the mechanism of projection as in paranoia, but of the (hysterical) hallucinatory mechanism. This shows one of its marked differentiations from paranoia. The other differentiation is to be found in the termination of dementia præcox. In general the outcome in the latter is more unfavorable than in paranoia. The victory does not remain in the reconstruction, as in paranoia, but in the repression. The regression not only goes as far as narcism and manifests itself as delusions of grandeur, but it proceeds to the complete abandonment of the object love and returns to the infantile autoerotism. The predisposed fixation therefore must lie further back than the one in paranoia. It must exist in the beginning of development, striving from autoerotism to object love. Like so many others Freud considers the term dementia præcox awkward. He also objects to Bleuler's designation of Schizophrenia.

He contends that the latter term appears right only when one does not think of its verbal significance and that it is too prejudicial inasmuch as it makes use of a theoretically postulated character which does not belong exclusively to the affection and, in the light of other views cannot be considered as the essential one. He proposes the name paraphrenia, the indefinite content of which expresses its relation to paranoia and hebephrenia.

References

1. Jahrbuch für Psychoanalytische u. Psychopathologische Forschungen, Bleuler-Freud, Vol. III.

2. Ueber die Rolle der Homosexualität in der Pathogenese der Paranoia, *l. c.*, p. 101; also, Reizung der Analen erogenen Zonen als auslösende Ursache der Paranoia, Zentralblatt für Psychoanalyse, August, 1911.

3. Psychologische Untersuchungen an Dementia Præcox, *l. c.*, Vol. II, 1910. Similar conclusions have been reached by K. Abraham, in reference to Dementia præcox: Die psychosexuellen Differenzen der Hysterie und der Dementia Præcox, Zentralblatt für Nervenheilkunde und Psychiatrie, July, 1908.

4. Eine Kindheitserrinerung des Leonardo da Vinci. Schriften zur angewandten Seelenkunde, 1910, No. 7.

5. Ein Fall von multipler Perversion mit hysterischen Obszenen, Jahrbuch für Psychoanalytische und Psychopathologische Forschungen, II, 1910.

6. Paraphrased from Freud, *l. c.*

7. *Cf.* Abraham and Maeder, *l. c.*

8. The Interpretation of Dreams, p. 126. The Macmillan Co., New York.

9. *Cf.* Chap. IX.

10. *Cf.* Ferenczi: Introjection und Uebertragung, Jahrbuch für Psychoanal. und Psychopatholog. Forschungen, 1910, Vol. I; also Jones: The Action of Suggestion in Psychotherapy, Journal of Abnormal Psychology, Dec., 1910.

11. Paraphrased from Freud, *l. c.*

12. Freud: *L. c.*, p. 64.

CHAPTER VII

PSYCHOPATHOLOGY OF EVERY-DAY LIFE

Freud's Conception of Consciousness, Unconscious and Foreconscious

"Men's little ways are usually more interesting and often more instructive than their grand manners. When they are off guard they frequently show to better advantage than when they are on parade." —Dr. Henry Van Dyke.

In my discussion of the dream and the psychoneurotic mechanisms I have attempted to show that they are the result of psychic streams of contrary tendencies, each striving for expression, the ultimate outcome of which is a compromise between the two. Each has to make concessions, thus meeting each other half way and the result of this mutual accommodation is then a dream or a psychoneurotic symptom which represents the fulfilment of a wish. These mechanisms are not conscious, but rather unconscious processes. Unconscious, according to Freud, are all those psychic manifestations of which the person is unconscious. He actually does not discover them and they can only be brought to the surface by analysis. The unconscious is made up of the repressed material, that is, it consists of the sum total of those psychic processes which have been relegated to the depths of the unconscious from the very beginning of childhood. Thus all the primitive impulses that have been curbed and inhibited with the development of the individual are in a state of repression. They form points of crystalization for the later repressions which mainly consist of erotic material. The later experiences are naturally not subjected to the same amount of repression as the earlier and more primitive ones, hence some of them may remain in what Freud calls the foreconscious. As shown above the dream is the function of two separate systems. One subjects the activity of the other to a critique which results in an exclusion from consciousness. The criticizing system is in closer relation with consciousness than the one criticized. The former, the foreconscious, stands like a screen between the unconscious and consciousness. Both are unconscious in the psychological sense, but the unconscious is incapable of consciousness, while the foreconscious can reach consciousness after it fulfils certain conditions regarding censorship. It is the latter that directs our waking life and determines our voluntary conscious actions. Consciousness, as such, plays a very small part and is conceived by Freud as a sensory organ for the perception of psychic qualities. The repressed material or the unconscious consists of wishes which are always active and reach for expression whenever they have an opportunity to unite with an emotion from conscious life. They thus determine all our actions, and our character is mainly based on memory traces of those impressions that have influenced us most strongly—those of our early youth which almost never become conscious.

As we pointed out above the later repressions are made up of thoughts that are painful and intolerable which are intentionally crowded out of consciousness. The individual intentionally strives to forget them and he manifestly succeeds. This is a protective mechanism for the good of the organism, for what would happen to us if we were always confronted by the numberless painful and disagreeable incidents of life? However, what we imagine to be forgotten remains in the unconscious in a repressed state and forms a complex. The complex remains in an inert state until incited by some association. Thus, an elderly woman experiences a feeling of uneasiness whenever she by chance sees a red-haired person. She is unable to account for it, and of late it has especially annoyed her because one of the members of her club happens to be of the Titian type. Analysis showed that forty-eight years ago she had a very unpleasant experience with a red-haired schoolmate. She was not at all cognizant of this incident each time she felt that "sense of uneasiness" and was wont to attribute it to the popular prejudice. But as she considers herself above such prejudice she could not understand her rude manners toward the woman of the Titian type. It was only after a lengthy analysis, after all the resistances were broken, that the original incident became conscious to her.

These resistances are always active and only during sleep do they partially slacken. It is then that the repressed material comes to the surface in the form of dreams, but as the resistances never lose their full power, they distort everything that passes them to such an extent that the dreamer cannot recognize his repressed thoughts or his unattainable wishes. But it is not only in the abnormal states and in the dream that the repression fulfils wishes. We find that the same influences are also evinced in our waking states in psychopathological actions of every-day life.

By psychopathological actions we understand those incorrect psychic activities which the individual daily performs, but of which he is not conscious at the time being. Among these different manifestations may be mentioned lapses of memory, of talking, writing, mistakes, etc.[1]

Among the lapses of memory we may have the common occurrences of forgetting names, of forgetting words in poetry or foreign words. In all these cases we must first assume that the person in question does not suffer from any nervous or mental affection producing qualitative or quantitative memory disturbances and that the things forgotten have once been well known. Everyone is familiar with the feeling of being unable to recall a name or a word. We think of a person whose name we knew well, but try as hard as we may the name cannot be recalled. We see the person in our mind's eye. We think of hundreds of incidents and associations connected with him, but despite that his name cannot be recalled. Often other names occur to us which we immediately recognize as false, yet they persist in thrusting themselves into our minds. This may continue for hours or days until the correct name comes unexpectedly or we ask someone for it. We never think of the cause of our forgetting because it is so self-evident nor do we try to find why we suddenly recalled this long-sought-for name or word.

Freud tells us that the reason for this forgetting is, in many cases, due to its direct or indirect association with something repressed—that is, something disagreeable or painful. This has been fully confirmed by such observers as Bleuler, Jung, Riklin, Maeder and Jones. Personally I can state that in every case amenable to analysis I could corroborate Freud's observation. The following examples will serve as illustrations:

I. FORGETTING OF NAMES

(*a*) A young newspaper man to whom I explained Freud's ideas concerning the forgetting of names insisted that this could not be true and to prove his assertion he related the following incident:

"My friend Jack left the city recently and the other day I wrote him a letter. On addressing the envelope I failed to remember his surname. I began with 'Jack' and for the life of me I could not proceed. After at least five minutes thinking I finally recalled that his surname was Murphy. Now as he is my best friend I fail to see the disagreeable or painful connection." I then proceeded to analyze it by the "continuous association" method. I asked him to concentrate his mind on the word Murphy and tell me all the associations it evoked. He produced the following: "Murphy recalls my friend Jack. We went to school together and have been friends since." He then continued to give a number of incidents connected with their school life, all of which were of a rather pleasant nature and added: "You see, I could talk about Jack and myself for hours." Asked whether he knew any other Murphy he was at first pretty sure that he did not, but he soon recalled his friend's brother for whom he entertained great regard. After awhile he recalled another Murphy, Mr. Murphy, of Tammany fame. He dislikes Tammany Hall and its leader "as every good Republican does, but that is no reason for forgetting Jack's name." He then continued to associate freely from one idea to another until he suddenly broke into laughter and then remarked: "It is funny that I did not think of it before. I now remember another Murphy, a newspaper man whom I know very well." Asked to tell something about him he said:" This is the only man I hate" and then delivered a long tirade against this Mr. Murphy.

We can now understand why he could not recall his friend's name. The name Murphy was under repression because it represented a person whom he hated. His own friend's name was also Murphy, but to him it was always Jack. He always called him Jack and in his mind it was Jack and not Murphy. He never corresponded with him before. This was the first time he was obliged to use Jack's surname. He could not recall it (1) because it was directly connected with something unpleasant to him and (2) he could not resign himself to give Jack the name of the man he hated.

The last mechanism is often observed in such slips of the tongue as the following: While conversing Mrs. S., inquiring about a mutual friend, said: "How is Mrs. Brown?" She was immediately corrected by a "You mean Mrs. Blank" to which she replied "Yes, Mrs. Blank. I made a mistake." There was only one reason, I thought, why she called Mrs. Blank by her maiden name which was Brown and to test my theory I said: "What is wrong with Mr. Blank?" She thoughtlessly answered "Oh, I don't like him," and then becoming conscious of what she said she showed her embarrassment by blushing, but she added consciously "I never liked him; I am sorry she married him."

Here the mistake showed her dislike for Mr. Blank. The repression fulfills her wish in not recognizing the marriage by continuing to use the maiden name. It is of quite different significance, however, if the lady herself continues to use her maiden name after marriage. Freud mentions the case of a lady who years before her divorce continued to use her maiden name in signing documents, etc.

(*b*) While reading one day the text recalled to me a case which I had published years before. I desired to make a marginal note to that effect when I suddenly found that I could not recall the name of my patient. This patient was under my personal care for months and the features of the case were such that I had daily spent hours with him, so that it was the more remarkable that I could not recall the name. As usual I made a great effort to recall it and it was only after some time that I thought of Freud's theories and decided to test them by analyzing this lapse of memory. The case had presented so many unusual and interesting aspects that I was advised to publish it. After a painstaking preparation I was ready to send it to the publisher when I was informed that my senior had decided to read a paper on this very subject before a medical society and that I was to have this paper ready for him on a certain date. My feelings on hearing this can readily be imagined. The thought of having labored for days and of some one else getting the credit for it caused me indignation and depression. My colleagues sympathized with me, but all they could do was to make merry over it. This continued until the day before the meeting when I was informed that owing to unforseen circumstances I was to attend this meeting myself and read the paper. I read this paper as directed, but very few of the members knew the true circumstances of the matter. Most of them thought that I was merely sent to read the paper. The reports of the meeting as given in the different medical journals gave the name of my senior as the reader of the paper. The reader will pardon my indulging in personalities. It is indispensable in psychanalysis and here it serves to show the marked displeasure and pain which caused the repression.

When one attempts to follow Freud's method of "free association" he soon finds himself in a maze. The longer he proceeds the more complicated the problem seems to become and to the inexperienced it appears like an endless confusion. Now and then our thoughts, as it were, stop. We call this an "obstruction" or a "blocking" and experience teaches us that this phenomenon generally accompanies or precedes some important complex. In analyzing psychoneurotic symptoms the patients often stop and say "That's all. I cannot think of anything else." After considerable urging they finally, perhaps after blushing, laughing or stammering, do think of something else. Frequently the mind makes use of symbolic expressions and ambiguous terms which the physician must always be alive to. All these are due to the inhibitions of the psychic censor against the painful and disagreeable thoughts.

On beginning to discover by analysis the name of my patient I soon found myself in a very complicated *milieu*. I distinctly saw his features in my mind. I reviewed all the circumstances connected with the case and noted all my associations. Page after page was filled and time flew faster than it seemed. I suddenly found that I had spent five hours of assiduous application and filled over two dozen pages, but was seemingly as far from getting the name as when I first started. Frequently my thoughts stopped only to start anew. I was most desirous not only of recalling the name, but of testing Freud's theory, as it was my first attempt. It would be useless and impossible to recall the different associations, but the following will suffice to explain the analysis: On seeing the patient in my mind's eye the name Appenzeller presented itself to me. Appenzeller was one of my patients in the psychiatrical clinic at Zurich where I was at the time of the analysis. There was no resemblance between the two patients except that my New York patient was a psychic epileptic and Appenzeller suffered from motor epilepsy, yet the latter name persistently emerged from the association mass. The scenes connected with my New York patient as well as numerous other hospital experiences continued to pass in a panoramic review. Some were especially persistent and vivid, recurring with greater frequency than the others. Thus, one scene, an actual occurrence, was especially vivid. It recalled a forest fire near the hospital. I stood watching the fire with my senior, Dr. Z., who played such a great part in the episode, and Dr. X. joined me. Many rabbits driven out by the fire were shot. While thus standing Dr. Z. turned to a hospital attendant and asked him for his shotgun as a rabbit was seen running from the underbrush. He waited for the animal to come within range and then got ready to fire, remarking: "Let me see whether I can get this rabbit." A crack was heard, but the rabbit scampered away. Dr X. and I looked at each other smilingly, but quickly changed countenance when Dr. Z. turned to us and said "My finger slipped on account of the rain." This scene persistently recurred from time to time, but I attached no more weight to it than to the hundreds of others. Yet whenever my supply of associations seemed to be exhausted and I started over again, the name of Appenzeller and this scene continually reappeared. I finally tired of the whole process and thought of giving it up, but despite my willingness to do so I could not banish the numerous scenes from my mind. While thus contemplating I again saw the rabbit scene and heard Dr. Z. say, "Let me see whether I can get this rabbit," and just then the name of the patient suddenly came to me. It was "Lapin" which is the French for rabbit.

It can readily be seen that had I been keen enough it would have saved me hours of labor for during the analysis this scene occurred twenty-eight times more than any other. But owing to my inexperience at the time and my intense desire to get the name I overlooked the very thing Freud lays so much stress upon—that is, the symbolic expressions, etc. This whole rabbit scene symbolizes the Lapin episode. Dr. Z. attempted to get the rabbit (Lapin) but missed it. To be sure, it must be remembered that although I am conversant with French, in my mind Lapin was always translated into rabbit because I think in English. In fact I distinctly recall that I had frequently translated mentally the name Lapin into rabbit. If we now bear in mind the French pronunciation of Lapin we can understand why Appenzeller continued to substitute itself. The first part—Appen—phonetically resembles Lapin—Appen, Lapen. Furthermore, both patients suffered from epilepsy. The case clearly shows how a name may be repressed on account of a disagreeable experience.

(*c*) A colleague who was acquainted with Freud's theories asked me to help him recall the name of one of his patients whom he treated almost daily for three months up to five weeks before he spoke to me. He was thinking of him on his way to see me and was surprised to have forgotten the name. Analysis gave the following associations: "He is a broker who was once well to do. For three months he was under my care. I cured him of a grave illness. He has not paid me for treatment, though he promised long ago to do so. The last time he came to see me he wanted me to sign some papers for him which I refused to do as I did not care to make any false statements. Since then I have not heard from him. It now occurs to me that the name ends with 'son.'" He then gave a number of names ending with "son" all of which he recognized as incorrect. Again the patient's ingratitude. "When I cured him he was grateful. He kept on saying that he would never forget what I had done for him and that as soon as he returned to business he would pay me what he owed me"—sudden blocking—then recalled his own ingratitude. He, too, is under obligations to a distant relative whom he dislikes, but to whom he owes much. He received a letter six weeks before, requesting the loan of a sum of money, but after reading it he mislaid it and never thought of it again. His relative's name is Brown—suddenly recalls his former patient's name "Bronson."

Here the forgetfulness was determined not so much by his patient's action as by the disagreeable feeling connected with his own affair. He was under obligations to Mr. Brown. He really should have sent him the money requested but "times are bad" and, strange to say, he mislaid the letter and never thought of it. In this connection it may be mentioned that this is the usual mechanism of mislaying. Things which we really value we never mislay.

(*d*) A man was urged by his wife to attend a social function in which he not only took no interest, but which he was sure would actually bore him. Yielding to his wife's entreaties he began to take his dress suit from the trunk when he suddenly thought of shaving. After accomplishing this he returned to the trunk and found it locked. Despite a long, earnest search, the key could not be found. A locksmith could not be found on Sunday evening so that the couple had to send their regrets. On having the trunk opened the next morning the lost key was found within. The husband had absentmindedly dropped the key into the trunk and sprung the lock. He assured me that this was wholly unintentional and unconscious. It must, however, be borne in mind that he did not wish to go. There was a motive, as we see, in the mislaying. A lover never misplaces a letter from his sweetheart nor does he ever mislay or forget to mail a letter written to her. We only mislay what we do not want. We are more apt to mislay letters containing bills than checks.

(*e*) The same mechanism comes into play in the missending of letters. One of my patients was corresponding with a woman to whom he was favorably disposed. One day he received a letter from her which, on opening, he found was meant for another man who was also one of her admirers. In this letter she refused a proposal made by the latter. The mistake served to show my patient that he was not her only admirer and thus stirred him to greater activities. At the same time it showed the other fellow why he was rejected as the letter which he received and which was meant for my patient was a very amorous epistle.

II. FORGETTING A RESOLUTION IS DUE TO SIMILAR CAUSES

(*a*) While absorbed in reading S. interrupted himself, opened a box containing numerous books, pamphlets and papers and began to rummage through them. He soon stopped, however, not knowing what he was looking for. He was sure that he wanted something from the box, but he could not recall what it was. He looked over many things, but did not recognize what he wanted. On trying to recall the motive for opening the box he was attracted by the open book which he left on the table and then thought that there must have been something in what he was just reading which caused him to open the box. With this in view he began to re-read the page and plainly recalled its contents as far as he had read, the last sentence being, "We feel more than we know." It was while thinking of this sentence that he stopped and opened the box. On freely associating to this last sentence he obtained the following: "We feel more than we can ever know. I feel that I ought to marry, but I do not know whether I really should. I used to feel that my fiancée did not really love me, but, as a matter of fact, I was not sure of it. I worried much over it, but it was merely a lover's doubt. I am now sure of her love. She wants to marry as soon as I return and wishes to have an elaborate church wedding which I dislike. But perhaps that will not come to pass. Something might happen. I have recently read of the stormy seas. An accident might happen to me while crossing the ocean," (feeling of fear and jealousy) and the thought "after all I may also be a specter bridegroom" suddenly recalled that he had been looking for Washington Irving's "Sketch Book."

This incident occurred while S. was abroad and his fiancée was in the United States. While abroad he was asked to translate for a foreign periodical a short story from English literature and he selected the Specter Bridegroom from Washington Irving's "Sketch Book." The day before the incident recounted above he had received a letter from the editor of the *Revue* telling him that under separate cover he was sending the proof sheets of the translation for correction. He thought of looking for the "Sketch Book" which he had in the box, but failed to do so just then. It was while unconsciously ruminating over the above cited sentence that the Specter Bridegroom came to his mind and he set out to find it, but as he unconsciously identified himself with Count von Altenberg, the unfortunate hero of Irving's sketch, who was killed while on his way to his bride, the painful thought was quickly repressed, taking with it all the concomitant associations.

(*b*) A confrère tells me the following experience: He started to make a call on a patient in a certain street, but instead of going there he called upon another patient. The reason for this was very simple. Patient number one paid his bill every January, while patient number two paid for each visit. That morning the doctor was in need of money, hence he would have preferred to go to patient number two.

(*c*) One of my patients, a music teacher, told me a

similar experience. On going to see a pupil in New York City he unexpectedly landed in Brooklyn. The music teacher carried on a secret love affair with his pupil's sister, and was accustomed to see her every evening after the lesson. He usually gave the lesson in the evening, but this time he was told to come in the morning. He knew well that he would not see her in the morning because she would be at work, but de did not like to refuse lest it might arouse suspicion. On going to give the lesson he simply rode too far, "having been absorbed in his newspaper." As it was too late to return from Brooklyn and give the lesson in the morning he was forced to postpone it till the evening. He assured me that he really intended to go to his pupil's house.

(*d*) Another patient invited two ladies to spend an evening at the theater. It was decided by the ladies to see the play "Alias Jimmy Valentine." On getting into the cab he unconsciously ordered the driver to take them to another theater and did not notice his mistake until they arrived at the wrong theater. Then it was too late to rectify it. Here it was the case of a homosexual person who was in constant fear of the law and who disliked to see a play dealing with convicts and prisons. The theater to which he ordered the driver to take him presented the play "The Three Daughters of Mons. Dupont," which deals with a selfish father who was finally brought to reason by his own children. He disliked his own father and was constantly trying to show him how to live properly. His mistakes served to exchange a disagreeable for an enjoyable evening.

These examples show that forgetting a resolution is

exactly the same as forgetting to recall a name or word —that is, it is always determined by a painful motive.

III. MISTAKES IN SPEAKING, READING AND WRITING

Mistakes in speaking show a similar mechanism. The disturbing influence is either a single unconsciously remaining thought which manifests itself through the mistake and can often be discovered only after detailed analysis, or it is a general psychic motive directed against the whole thing spoken.

(*a*) At a private theatrical rehearsal the hero, instead of saying "I love you, Emma," said "I love you, Helen." The latter was the name of the girl with whom he was really in love.

(*b*) Recently an acquaintance asked me to introduce him to one of my friends who was about to leave for Europe. I did not like to do it, but I could not possibly refuse. After hesitating for awhile I said "Come around next Sunday and I'll take you to his office." My wife, who was near, interposed with "Why, he sails Saturday." I immediately corrected myself, saying "I meant Friday." Here the mistake was the answer to the thought, "I wonder how I can avoid this." Fortunately my acquaintance knew nothing of Freud's mechanisms.

(*c*) A lady, talking about her husband with whom she lived a very unhappy life because he was addicted to drink, said among other things, "I can never discuss with him any intelligent topic because he is so full," meaning "dull."

(*d*) A friend described to me a nervous patient and wished me to know whether I could benefit him. I remarked "I believe that in time I could remove all his symptoms by psychanalysis because it is a durable case," wishing to say "curable." It was not merely the sound association between the two words which caused the mistake. From the description I diagnosed the case as chronic hysteria and experience teaches that such cases generally require a very protracted treatment, hence durable.

(*e*) A young man, talking about an old woman who was foolishly in love with him, said "I am thinking seriously of burying her" instead of marrying. Here the lapsus linguæ betrays his inner feelings in the matter. He would marry this old and wealthy woman if he should know that she would soon die and leave him her money.

(*f*) While walking one night with a friend we accidentally met a colleague, Dr. P. whom I had not seen for years and of whose private life I knew nothing. We were naturally very pleased to meet again and on my invitation he accompanied us to a café where we spent about two hours in pleasant conversation. To my question as to whether he was married he gave a negative answer and added, "Why should a man like me marry?"

On leaving the café he suddenly turned to me and said: "I should like to know what you would do in a case like this. I know a nurse who was named as co-respondent in a divorce case. The wife sued the husband for divorce and named her as co-respondent and he got the divorce." I interrupted him saying "You mean she got the divorce." He immediately corrected himself, saying, "Yes, she got the divorce" and continued to tell how the excitement of the trial had affected this nurse to such an extent that she became nervous and took to drink. He wanted me to advise him how to treat her, etc.

As soon as I corrected his mistake I asked him to explain it, but, as is usually the case, he was surprised at my question. He wanted to know whether a person had no right to make mistakes in talking. I explained to him that there is a reason for every mistake and that if he had not told me that he was unmarried I would say that he was the hero of the divorce case in question and that the mistake showed that he wished he had obtained the divorce instead of his wife; so as not to be obliged to pay the alimony and to be permitted to marry again in New York City. He stoutly denied my interpretation, but his emotional agitation, followed by loud laughter, only strengthened my suspicions. To my appeal that he should tell the truth for science sake, he said "Unless you wish me to lie you must believe that I was never married and hence your psychanalytic interpretation is all wrong." He, however, added that it was dangerous to be with a person who paid attention to such little things. Then he suddenly remembered that he had another appointment and left us.

Both my friend and I were convinced that my interpretation of his lapsus linguæ was correct and I decided to corroborate or disprove it by further investigation. The next day I found a neighbor, an old friend of Dr. P., who confirmed my interpretation in every particular. The divorce was granted to Dr. P.'s wife a few weeks before and a nurse was named as co-respondent. A few weeks later I met Dr. P. and he told me that he was thoroughly convinced of the Freudian mechanisms.

(*g*) A homosexual whom I treated for some time and who considered himself cured made this mistake on leaving my office: instead of saying "I shall now go to the Hotel Robespierre" he said, "I shall now go to the Hotel St. Pierre." I noticed his mistake and asked him whether he knew of a hotel in New York City by the name of St. Pierre. He stated that he had never heard of a hotel named the St. Pierre and that he meant to say the Hotel Robespierre.

The analysis furnished the following associations: "St. Pierre—St. Peter—Rome—adoration,"—he recalled having seen the devout kiss the toe of St. Peter while he was in the Cathedral at Rome—from Rome he went to Pompei where he saw some remnants of the old phallic worship—the big toe recalled one of his phallic symbols (as a child he was a toe sucker)—he then thought of fellatio which, he said, no longer had any attraction for him as he was now heterosexual and very pleased over it—he then stopped and again thought of St. Peter and Rome and said: "They stand for the old order of things, strict adherence to the old orthodox religion—they are against all reforms—Robespierre reminds me of revolution, complete change of the order of things, including religion—they stopped worshipping Christ and worshipped instead the Goddess of Reason, a woman of questionable reputation."

His stock of associations was exhausted and I did not urge him to continue as I could now interpret his mistake in speaking. When he was about to leave my office he intended to visit his mistress who lived in the Hotel Robespierre. His mistake showed his unconscious resistance against heterosexuality. He would still prefer to cling to the "old order of things," of worshipping the man rather than the woman.

(*h*) My traveling companion, who for some reason, took particular pleasure in railing at the medical profession, remarked once, "The most appropriate name for a doctor I ever heard of I read in this morning's Sun. It was Dr. Slayers, etc." I became interested and asked him to show me the article and to his surprise the name was not Slayers, but Salyers. Here his unconscious thought "Doctors are butchers" took advantage of the close similarity of the words and caused this metathesis.

(*i*) A young bride who was obliged to remain at home on Sunday morning and transcribe her husband's manuscript instead of attending church, as was her custom, wrote *Bridle* March instead of *Bridal* March and *parson* instead of *person*.

(*j*) On re-reading an abstract which I made from a foreign journal I was surprised to find that instead of writing "Markuse even went so far as to recommend sexual intercourse as a therapeutic agent for unmarried women" I wrote "the great Markuse, etc." I then recalled that while reading about Markuse's very bold recommendation I was most surprised and said to myself "Such courage could only be evinced by either a very great or an eccentric man" and knowing the scientific attainments of Markuse I readily eliminated the second part of the postulate. Having decided that he was a great man my unconscious thought found it easy to produce by metathesis from *Markuse* the Greek word *Makros* (long, big, great).

Mistakes in printing are of a similar nature. As a

classical example of this type may be cited the "Wicked Bible" so-called from the fact that the negative was left out of the Seventh Commandment. This authorized edition of the Bible was published in London in 1631 and it is said that the printer had to pay a fine of two thousand pounds for the ommission.

IV. SYMBOLIC ACTIONS

Symbolic actions, according to Freud, are those performances which a person does unconsciously and automatically and which he considers as meaningless, indifferent and accidental when his attention is called to them. Such actions, depending on their determinations, are either simple or complicated and manifest themselves in either such insignificant acts as scribbling aimlessly with one's lead pencil, jingling the coins in one's pocket, kneading of soft substances, etc., or in more complicated acts. All such performances generally conceal sense and meaning for which any other outlet is closed.

Symbolic or accidental actions can be observed both among normal and abnormal persons. They are of special interest to the doctor who finds many valuable hints for the interpretation of symptoms and to the student of human nature to whom they tell volumes. The popular saying "actions speak louder than words" is especially true of the manifestly insignificant and accidental ones. Such actions often refer to a person's complexes—that is, to a complex of ideas of strong feeling tone which show a tendency to become split off from consciousness and repressed into the unconscious. We are wont to look at everything under the guise of a particular complex. Thus the misreading of Slayer for Salyer is an example of complex constellation. This gentleman had some unpleasant experiences with a doctor, hence the misreading is merely a symbolic expression of his repressed complex. Such complex symbols are expressed in peculiar complicated acts. Jung cites the case of a young lady who "when promenading wished to take along a baby carriage. The reason for this, as she blushingly admitted, was because she desired to be looked upon as married. I know an old maid who wears a wedding ring, especially when traveling. Her reason for wearing it is "because it was my grandmother's. Other examples of symbolic actions are the following:

(*a*) A woman song writer and poet who led a very unhappy life continued to write on the happiness of matrimony and just before she obtained a divorce she gave out a song entitled "How to Keep a Husband." Another writer on "The Home Beautiful" recently asked the court to divorce her from her husband.

(*b*) A noted artist and writer of sonnets on the happiness of perfect marriage forsook his first wife for an affinity, maltreated his second wife, for which he was arrested and punished, and now that he is finally divorced, he is going through similar experiences with a third wife.

(*c*) The patient mentioned before, while despairing of his life because he imagined himself afflicted with an incurable disease, continued to occupy himself with Ibsen's "When We Dead Awaken."

(*d*) A New York embezzler who was discovered by detectives in a Philadelphia public library was found reading a book entitled "Will I ever go Back?"

(*e*) The selection of Washington Irving's Spectre Bridegroom for translation in the aforementioned example is another symbolic action of this kind. Selections of certain professions are usually symbolic actions. Thus I know an actress and a lawyer who are very bad stutterers. Here the professions serve to conceal the real defect, for no one would ever think that an actress or a lawyer could lack the most essential requirement of their callings.

When I became interested in this question I asked some of my confrères how they came to study medicine and I received very interesting answers of which I will mention two. Dr. W. stated that since his early youth he thought of studying medicine. As an infant, he became afflicted with infantile paralysis, the effects of which he still shows, and as the doctors could not help him he thought of finding a cure himself. Dr. B. could give no definite reason, but finally recalled that when he was very young he overheard a conversation between his mother and another woman. The latter asked his mother in what month he was born and on being told that it was October she dryly remarked "He will be either a doctor, a butcher or a murderer. He will have to shed blood." As he did not care to adopt the last two professions he became a doctor. Some may think that the compromise includes them all. I can definitely assert that in this case it was an unconscious process.

It is interesting to see what part such symbolic actions play in every-day life.

(*a*) A young married woman asked her husband for money to make some purchases on their way home. While talking she suddenly threw away the ten dollar bill as though it were a valueless piece of paper. Her husband noticed it and picked it up without her perceiving it. Not until she reached the store did she notice that she had lost the bill. This woman was wont to contribute ten dollars monthly to a charitable society before her marriage. While promenading she spoke to her husband about it and he said that it would be best to stop it for the time being, to which she had to acquiesce. It was after this conversation that she threw away the bill. This action was the equivalent of the thought "You do not allow me to give it to charity so I throw it away so that some poor person may find it." That is, it was meant as a sacrifice.

(*b*) A woman continued to oversalt everything she cooked for her husband. At the same time she persistently forgot to place salt on the table. By this she meant to express "I am in love, but you are not." For it is said that when a woman is in love she oversalts the food. In fact she always talked of her husband's indifferences and her ardent love.

Some symbolic actions continue to manifest themselves for long periods, sometimes for life, and are considered personal characteristics of the individual evincing them. Such activities are very often only reactions of some repressed impulses and are either the symbolic expressions of the repressed wishes or represent contrasts of the same. A good example of the last type is the woman mentioned before who insisted upon paying cash for everything. Another example of this kind was a young man of twenty-eight years who was very religious and over-scrupulous in everything. In fact his relatives and intimate friends considered him "a bit too religious and over-conscientious." Examination showed that his outward expression of piety and conscientiousness was a contrast manifestation of his unconscious. For years he had been struggling with sexual temptations. He saw sex where no one else did. He went through the usual conflicts of the masturbator, the struggles against illicit sex and finally thought he was victorious. For two years before he came to me, he led what he called "a pure life." He shunned the society of women and his moral sensitiveness verged on eccentricity. A few examples obtained from himself will show his personality. When a woman addressed him and asked to be directed to a certain street he turned his head away from her fearing that she might arouse sex fancies. He was once present at a social gathering at which a dispute arose between a young man and a young woman as to who was the taller of the two. To settle this they stood back to back and asked the others to express judgment. He became excited over this and left the room. He thought that their action was immoral. Yet while he was an ardent member of the church and was held up as a model young man he spent hours in disreputable neighborhoods. In fact his time was divided between the church and the slums. To be sure his object in frequenting these places was "to do good." He wished "to eradicate the canker that eats its way into innocent minds." To effect this he would allow himself to be accosted by prostitutes and then have them arrested. On a few occasions he really yielded to temptation which naturally increased his zeal for "eradicating the canker." In reality, however, he did all these things because he unconsciously desired them and his every-day piety was a symbolic contrast expression.

Symbolic actions of long duration which are the direct results of repressed wishes furnish a wide field for collecting-manias or peculiar hobbies. I do not refer to those who confine their activities to the collection of valuable or scientific objects such as books, paintings, etc., but I mean those persons who collect things without any definite aim, who can give no reason for their activity and whose collections as such are of no scientific value. I can best explain what I mean by giving the following examples:

(*a*) An unmarried woman of thirty-six years took a great interest in mushrooms. She not only took her vacation during the mushroom season so as to be able to study and gather them, but she also collected many works on the subject, especially those containing colored charts. She had no scientific interest in the subject and could give no reason for her action. She only knew that mushrooms fascinated her. Analysis showed that she began to take an interest in mushrooms a few years before while she was on her vacation. She passed a restless night, having been troubled by many nightmares. While taking a walk early in the morning she found some mushrooms. This was the beginning of her interest in mushrooms. Further investigation showed that at the time she resisted many sexual temptations which would also account for her insomnia and nightmares.[2] The interest for mushrooms was aroused by their resemblance to the penis. Phallus is the scientific name for some species of mushrooms.

(*b*) Some years ago while traveling in Europe I happened to be in the same railroad compartment with a western gentleman. He was a hail-fellow-well-met so we soon became acquainted. He was a man of means who was traveling for his health and discovering that I was a physician he soon became confidential. He told me that he was suffering from a nervous disease and asked me to recommend him some professor in Paris. We were together for about twelve hours and as we had to pass two boundary lines I noticed that he carried with him a small suit case which he guarded very carefully. It was filled with stick-pins of all descriptions which he bought as souvenirs in every European city of importance. To my remark that he must have a great many very good friends to buy for them so many stickpins he replied that they were not meant to be given away. He stated that he would not be foolish enough to give away so many valuable presents, but that he collected them for his pleasure. "Some people," he said, "when they travel collect pictures. I made up my mind to collect stickpins." He did not know just why he collected them. "I bought a few for myself," he said, "and then I just kept it up."

As I said before the man came to Europe to seek relief from a nervous trouble. When he asked me to recommend him some professor I was compelled to ask him to explain his ailment as I could not see anything organically wrong with him. He then told me that he has been suffering for years from psychic impotence and that he had consulted many specialists in the United States without obtaining any relief and that he met with no better success in Europe. He described his malady in the following words: "I have the desire and I have erections when I am alone, and sometimes I can even have an erection when I am with a woman, but I can't *stick* it in. When I try this the erection fades." May we not assume that his collection of stickpins was an unconscious activity to get that which he most desired in reality?

Music, too, is used to give expression to one's complexes. While doing some experimental work in the same laboratory with Dr. L. he continued to whistle for hours an old melody. It was the refrain from the old song "Don't Be Angry, that Cannot be." Having been acquainted with the contents of this song I wondered whether his mechanical whistling expressed the feeling of a rejected love. On asking him why he whistled so much he characteristically replied "I don't know myself." I then asked him whether he knew what he was whistling, but be assured me that he did not. "It is some street song," he said. "I have a habit of whistling while I work." I then told him the words and jokingly asked him whether he had been rejected by the girl he loved. He emphatically denied it, but his emotional reactions only strengthened my suspicion so that I continued my investigations. That evening we met at a café and after I had gained his confidence, he disburdened his heart. Only the evening before he had proposed and had been rejected.

These examples show that there is nothing arbitrary or fortuitous in our actions. No matter how trivial or voluntary, analysis always shows that this action is fully determined by unconscious motives. Those who believe in a free will naturally dispute this theory, but it is always possible to demonstrate to their own satisfaction that whatever they consider a voluntary act done with a free will is nevertheless unconsciously determined by definite motives. One of my unbelieving patients forgot his umbrella in my office and then asked me to explain this forgetting. "Surely," he said, "I did not wish to lose a new umbrella." I fully agreed with him for if he wanted to lose it he would have left it elsewhere. He came to see me daily and as the rain ceased during his visit he could leave it until his next visit. Moreover, every psychanalyst knows that patients who are pleased with the treatment often forget things at the doctor's office. This simply means that they expect and wish to return. We never forget anything valuable where we do not wish to return. The same holds true for losing things. We never lose what we value highly and, everything being equal, whatever we lose we usually don't want. A distant relative of Prof. Freud, who on account of family jealousy, disputed his theories, spoke one day very disparagingly about his theory of wit. I observed that he had no conception of the subject in question and did not hesitate to tell him this. His excuse was that he could not read the whole book because he lost it. Here, of course, the losing was intentional. An excellent example of definite determinism is related by Dr. Ernest Jones. One of his unbelieving acquaintances produced the number 986 and defied him to connect it with anything of special interest in the mind. Jones made use of the free-association method and the acquaintance recalled the following associations: Six years before on a very hot day he had seen a joke in an evening newspaper which stated that the thermometer had stood 986° Fahrenheit, evidently an exaggeration of 98.6° Fahrenheit. Jones was curious to know why this memory had persisted with such vividness as to be so readily brought out, for with most persons it surely would have been forgotten beyond recall unless it became associated with some other mental experience of more significance. The next thought was the general reflection that the conception of heat had always greatly impressed him, that heat was the most important thing in the universe, the source of life and so on. Jones thought that the young man's prosaic attitude needed some explanation and he therefore pressed him for more associations. The next thought was of a factory stack which he could see from his bedroom window. He often stood watching the flame and smoke issuing out of it in the evening and reflecting on the deplorable waste of energy. "Heat, flame, the source of life, the waste of vital energy issuing from an upright hollow tube—it was not hard to divine from such associations that the ideas of heat and fire were unconsciously linked in his mind with the idea of love, as is so frequent in symbolic thinking, and that there was a strong masturbation complex present, a conclusion that he presently confirmed. His choice of a number was therefore far from being a free one, being in fact related to a very significant personal constellation."[3]

As an example of how one takes up innocent associations for the purpose of giving vent to one's complexes I will relate the following episode:

A husband read a joke in some periodical which struck him as being particularly funny so that he laughed heartily at it and then repeated it to his wife. The joke was something like this: Teacher (to class of boys): "Having more than one wife is polygamy. Now, Johnny, if a man has only one wife what would you call that?" Johnny: "Monotony." To the surprise of the husband his wife was not at all affected by the joke. Indeed she couldn't see why he laughed so much over it. A few days later while visiting a friend the conversation turned to the general topic of man's fickleness and so on. The wife wistfully remarked: "I know exactly in what channels Frank's (husband) mind runs" and to explain herself she repeated the aforementioned joke, but when she came to Johnny's answer she said "Monopoly" instead of "monotony."

The mistake here corrects the tendency of the joke. She disliked to hear her husband laugh over a joke the underlying thought of which was to the effect that one wife means monotony. She realized that his hearty laughter signified his agreement with the thought underlying the joke. It pained her to think that her husband should find her monotonous and laugh at a joke that suggested polygamy. Her mistake cleverly expressed her disapproval of the idea implied by the joke and at the same time shows in what she believed. She wanted a monopoly on her husband.

Such complex indicators expressed in every-day conversations and actions are not rare. The careful observer finds them everywhere. For nothing can be concealed. Repressed thoughts forever strive to come to the surface and just as the insane realize their ideals in their insanities, we realize our wishes through our dreams and in the "little ways" of every-day life.

References

1. Freud: Psychopathologie des Alltagsleben, 3d Ed., Karger, Berlin. English translation in preparation.

2. Jones: On the Nightmare, Am. Jour. of Insanity, Jan., 1910.

3. Jones: The Psychopathology of Every-day Life, Am. Jour. of Psychology, Vol. XXII.

CHAPTER VIII

HYSTERICAL FANCIES AND DREAMY STATES

When we enter into the deeper mental processes, especially into those of hysteria, we invariably come across the quaint yet familiar psychic mechanisms of fancies or day dreams. Freud tells us that fancy formation is common to both sexes and that the fancies represent wish gratifications emanating from privation and longing. Like dreams they serve to relieve the overburdened mind and to secure comfort not to be obtained in reality. They are called "day dreams" because they furnish the key for the understanding of night dreams.[1] The hysterical fancies are jealously hidden as they belong to the most intimate estates of personality. They are found in both normal and neurotic individuals, but it is in the latter that they obtain prominence in the formation of symptoms. I fully agree with Freud that all analyzable hysterical attacks prove to be involuntary incursions of day dreams. Such fancies may remain conscious or merge into the unconscious. In the latter case they may become pathogenic and express themselves in symptoms and attacks. Under favorable conditions it is possible for consciousness to grasp and bring to light such unconscious fancies. Freud relates that one of his patients whose attention was called to these fancies later narrated the following occurrence: While in the street she suddenly found herself in tears and reflecting over the cause of her weeping the fancy became clear to her. She fancied herself in delicate relationship with a musician famous in the city whom she did not know. In her fancy she bore him a child (she was childless); later he deserted her leaving her with the child in misery. At this stage of the romance she burst into tears.

Such unconscious fancies have either been unconscious from the first, having been formed in the unconscious, or, what is more usual, they were once conscious and then intentionally forgotten and repressed into the unconscious. Their content usually undergoes many transformations and the resultant symptom or attack is often a very distorted mechanism. Analysis shows that the unconscious fancies are intimately connected with the person's sexual life. They are identical with the fancy which led to sexual gratification during the period of masturbation. The masturbating act originally consists of two parts, the provocation of the fancy and the active performance of self gratification at its height. It is first autoerotic and undertaken for the pleasure obtained from an erogenous zone, but later it becomes blended with a wish presentation referring to the love object and serves for a partial realization of the situation in which this fancy culminates. If this masturbo-fantastic gratification remains undone, the fancy changes from a conscious to an unconscious one. If no other manner of sexual gratification occurs, that is, if the person remains an abstainer and does not succeed in fully sublimating his libido, the unconscious fancies become refreshed. They grow exuberantly and at least a fragment of their content forms into symptoms or attacks.

The hysterical symptoms are merely unconscious fancies brought to light by "conversion" and inasmuch as they are somatic expressions they are often taken from the spheres of the sexual feelings and motor innervation which originally accompanied the former still conscious fancy. The disuse of onanism is thus made retrogressive and the final aim of the whole morbid process, the restoration of the primary sexual gratification, though never attaining perfection, always comes near to it. When we analyze these unconscious fancies of hysterics we find that they contently correspond to the situations of gratification enacted by perverts consciously. Thus an hysterical woman of thirty years went through strange episodes lasting from a few hours to days and weeks. One of these attacks which recurred quite often manifested itself by extreme anxiety during which the patient was very restless and anxious. She acted as though she was terrified. She moaned and cried, uttering the words "virtue, doctor, heroine," and made continuous attempts to get out of the room. The attack was always followed by an hysterical paralysis and excruciating pain in her legs which lasted for a few days. At times the attacks were characterized by some variations, ending with the *arc de cercle*, but they were essentially as described. Analysis showed that she identified herself with Maupassant's Clochette who broke her leg by jumping out of a second story window when surprised with her cowardly lover during a tryst in a loft.[2]

These attacks came on first after some gossip about her former love affair was repeated to her and meant to show that the statements were false, or in other words, that like Clochette "she was a martyr and a noble soul." The words she muttered were those repeated by the doctor in the story who said of Clochette: "That was her only love affair and she died a virgin." The identification was determined by the following facts: She had a love affair lasting for about a year which terminated with the sudden disappearance of her fiancé. Some evil tongues had it that she was left in a delicate state and her mother thought seriously of asking the family physician to silence the gossip. When she became hysterical one of her symptoms was pain all over the body especially in her legs. It was during a rest cure that she read Maupassant's Clochette which readily took her fancy not because it showed a striking resemblance to her case, but because she wished to be like Clochette and be defended by her doctor. In the course of time this wish allied itself with other wishes and the whole thing was subjected to the influence of the psychic censor. That accounted for the different variations which as in dreams were produced by condensation, multiple identification and inversion of events, etc.[3] Thus the *arc de cercle* was simply an inversion of the position during coitus.

Another patient, Miss M., thirty-six years old, an hysteric with many degenerative trends, referred to me by Dr. Frederick Peterson, went through many minor and major attacks which were based on real and fancied experiences. Her main symptom was an astasia abasia which lasted for years. She could neither walk nor sit up for any length of time and was forced to remain in bed in a peculiar constrained attitude, her body forming an angle, her head and legs being raised high by many pillows. Analysis brought out the following facts: As a child she masturbated herself and other children and resorted to many coprophilic activities such as playing with urine and feces. This was followed by a marked repression which gave rise to extreme feelings of disgust and morality. This stage was followed by a failure in the repression and a return of the things repressed. She then evinced a polymorphous perverse sexuality and practised many coprophilic activities. She refused to empty her bowels for days and sometimes for over a week in spite of all medications. While taking a rest cure in a well-known sanatorium she made believe that she could not attend to her natural wants, causing thereby much worriment and alarm to the doctors and nurses. While they exerted all their efforts to alleviate her apparent distress she was stealing towels and used them as receptacles for her excretions. She secretly threw these out of the window or hid them in her room. Her fancies were very prolific and the material for them was furnished by both fiction and reality. She was an ardent reader and whatever appealed to her fancy was immediately taken up and elaborated into her complexes. Her imaginative but rather defective mind made no distinction between fact and fancy so that whatever was once a fancy based on something read or heard soon became to her an actual experience.

She often recalled the typical pseudologia phantastica. It was due to this that she accused every physician coming in professional contact with her of having sexual designs upon her. It was really comical to hear the accusations she brought against at least a dozen of our most reputable men in the medical profession. She stated that everyone of them wanted to make her his mistress. She had absolutely no reason to give for her belief and psychanalysis showed that they were merely suppressed wish-phantasies which came to the surface as outer perceptions. This is the usual mechanism of all hysterical accusations against doctors.

The more deeply I penetrated into the patient's unconscious the more I became convinced that almost every one of her symptoms and attacks was determined by some former fancy. She read some erotic story and identified herself with one of the characters, and then lived through the whole situation over and over again. As she was bisexual she often identified herself with the male character of the story and then lived through, as it were, his part. A recurrent episode of this nature was the following: She began with a period of exaltation during which she would be very talkative and vivacious. She would play the piano and act some part (she was once an actress), usually the part of a man. This would continue from an hour to a few days and would suddenly be interrupted by severe headaches, nausea with occasional vomiting and a marked aggravation of the pains in her groin, abdomen and legs which she called "the three-cornered stone pains." The analysis brought out the following facts: At a very early age her father, wishing to stop her from crying, once put his hand under her dress and pinched her bare buttock and legs. This was often repeated on similar occasions and always had its effect. She then became very sensitive in these regions. She could not tolerate the slightest pressure there and was always complaining of her shoes and stockings. On one of these occasions when her father impatiently asked her what ailed her she lied and said that the skin was rubbed off her foot. He forced her to remove her shoe in the presence of many strangers and as no abrasion was found she was very much humiliated. About the same time her mother once forced her to sleep with a young man because there were many guests in the house. She again received a psychic trauma in the same region. Added to this she has a rather high instep which serves to accentuate her sensitiveness in her legs and feet. All these traumas took place before the age of five years. At the age of puberty she attended a private school and one night she witnessed by chance a homosexual act between a teacher and a favorite pupil. Years later she was abnormally fond of X., a girl of her own age. It was about this time that she read Balzac's Droll Stories and was very much affected by one of them. It dealt with a gay cavalier who seduced an innocent girl. This story produced many erotic feelings and fancies which continued for months until one day she dressed in male attire and called on X. She made believe that she was doing this just for fun and was demonstrating to X. how well she could play the part of a gay cavalier. The demonstration ended with a gross homosexual episode between herself and X., and as the latter was at the time engaged to be married she became very remorseful and blamed M. for leading her into temptation, adding "How can I look John (fiancé) in the face?" This, in turn, caused reproach and self-accusation in M., who brooded over it for some time and gradually repressed it. The attack mentioned above appeared shortly thereafter. It represented a fragment of sexual activity which becomes quite transparent when we think of the episode with X.

Some fancies are pure fabrications constructed of the patient's wishes. Thus, an intelligent young woman of thirty years sent to me for treatment by Dr. Israel Strauss had one fancy which she lived through from time to time. She imagined herself married to a tall, handsome and very wealthy man. She had three children, the like of whom did not exist. She lived on a beautiful yacht and entertained only such people as she and her husband really liked. This state of blissful happiness existed for a few days during which she was happy and contented. Then the whole structure crumbled. Her husband and children died and she was left alone in terrible depression lasting for days. She assured me that her reactions were very vivid and real, being mindful, however, that it was only a fancy.

Besides these fancies we come across other strange psychic processes which are designated as hysterical dreamy states. They are not the protracted crepuscular episodes followed by partial or complete amnesia which were described by Ganser and others and often taken as psychic equivalents of motor epilepsy, but they represent these peculiar conditions so often observed in psychoneurotics which were first described by Löwenfeld[4] and later submitted to a thorough psychanalytic study by Abraham.[5] The characteristics of these states will be best described by recalling to you the familiar old fable which is said to have originated in India and passed from the Sanskrit versions with many variations into many languages. The story selected by me tells how an oriental glass vender sat cross legged with his basket of glassware in front of him. While wishing for purchasers he merged into the following reverie: "If I sell this whole basket of glass I shall have ten dinars. I will then buy glassware for the whole sum and when that is sold I shall have twenty dinars. I will then buy glass for twenty dinars and sell it for forty dinars. For this sum I shall again buy glassware and when that will be sold I shall be worth eighty dinars," etc. In his reverie he kept doubling his fortune until he was immensely rich. He bought enchanted palaces, lived in luxury and lavished fortunes. His fancies became more and more extravagant. He was very happy and elated when a slight movement suddenly reminded him of his basket and the thought flashed through his mind "What's the use of bothering with such worthless stuff?" And with that he kicked the basket over. The clanging of the broken glass interrupted his day dream and brought him back to himself.

Let us for a moment think of this story which, *si non è vero, è ben trovato,* and examine the different mental operations which enter into its formation. It shows the following fairly well defined stages: There is a first stage of fantastic exaltation, the content of which deals with the individual's hopes and aspirations. The glass vender is in a state of euphoria. From a poor man he is suddenly transformed into a man of wealth and his fortune is rapidly increasing. This is followed by a stage of dream-like withdrawal from reality. He is no longer controlled by logical judgment and reasoning. His fancies, therefore, run riot as it were. Everything is changed. It is like a dream where time, space and natural obstacles are absent. He amasses an enormous fortune and owns palaces, etc. In brief, he is no longer himself. This is followed by a very rapid third stage which is distinguished by a suspension of consciousness, an absent-mindedness during which there are no thoughts so to speak, and the whole episode is followed by depression characterized by anxiety with its concomitant manifestations.[6] I need hardly say that our hero must have been depressed on emerging from his revery.

In almost all the cases observed by me these three stages, which were originally described by Abraham,[7] could readily be distinguished, but I should like to add that the first stage is always preceded by a period of craving.

Without going into detailed histories I shall cite some of my own observations.

Case I.—I. C. was seen by me in the neurological department of the Vanderbilt Clinic in November, 1908. Among other things he complained of strange thoughts which interfered with his work. He stated that he was a weaver by trade and that for months he was hardly able to attend to his work. He explained that weaving required concentration of attention, as a great deal of counting had to be done and that a single mistake spoiled the work. His "foolish" thoughts would come in spite of all effort to keep them away. They absorbed his mind to an extent that he forgot his work and unconsciously stopped weaving and continued dreaming until aroused. As examples he gave a few experiences of the previous day, which, in his own words, read as follows: "I am working and unconsciously I begin to think what I should do if I had two thousand dollars. I start a shop and soon earn a lot of money because I oppress my employees. With the money thus gained I open a big factory and employ a lot of greenhorns whom I force to work long hours for very little pay. I enlarge my business. I have hundreds of people working for me. I become greater and greater . . . . . when I suddenly find myself crying because I have lost all my money in Wall Street."

"I marry a very nice girl. She is very much in love with me, but she is afraid of me. I am very tyrannical and brutal. She has to do what I tell her, otherwise I beat her. She cries and begs me not to kill her, but I pay no attention to her. I become more and more excited. I hardly know what I do when I suddenly wake up wringing my hands because she is dead."

He recited many more day dreams, but they were all of the same nature. They all dealt with wealth and murder.

Recalling Freud's saying that the contented individual does not indulge in fantasies I assumed that these dreamy states must represent some of the patient's wishes, and viewed superficially one may think that the first dreamy state corroborates this assumption. The patient is a poor weaver who believes himself oppressed by his employer and therefore dreams of changing places with his oppressor. His day dream is simply a realization of his wishes. But a number of questions arise as soon as we take a closer view of the subject. In the first place it cannot be said that it is really a wish realization as the money thus rapidly gained is as rapidly lost, leaving the patient unhappier than he was. It may also be asked why the patient is not satisfied with the everyday conscious day dreaming. Why do these dreamy states come in attacks? Why are they accompanied by complete oblivion to external impressions, especially at their height, and why does the patient perceive them as unreal and strange? Moreover, when we recall the second dream, we can no longer think of any wish realization, for the patient is single and is very much in love with his fiancée whom he wishes to marry.

From the study of dreams we have learned that no matter how absurd a dream may seem it nevertheless contains sense and meaning if we find its latent content, and that every dream, and for that matter every psychotic symptom, contains the hidden fulfilment of a repressed wish[8] which usually refers to the two great impulses, hunger and love. Freud has also shown that certain episodic manifestations of hysteria are simply substitutive gratifications for the abandoned masturbation,[9] and Abraham maintains that the same is true for the hysterical dreamy state. Let us see whether this is true in our patient.

I regret that I was unable to make a complete analysis of his case. The patient was a clinic one and, as often happens in such cases, the analysis had to be given up. Still the facts that I have obtained are sufficient to confirm the assumption that his dreamy states were substitutions for his masturbation. His history was, briefly, as follows:

I. C. was twenty-two years old and had masturbated on and off since the age of twelve. From a very early age he had been suffering from a mixed neurosis (anxiety hysteria and compulsion neurosis) which was due to many conflicts and repressions. At the age of seventeen years he consorted with women and masturbated excessively besides. He came to New York at twenty years of age and after that tried very hard to abstain from sexual indulgence, but often failed. At twenty-two years he fell in love and decided to lead a life of sexual abstinence until his marriage which was to take place in March, 1909. The sadistic day dreams described above came on after a few weeks of hard struggle. He was always given to day dreaming, but he himself sharply distinguished between his former air castles and his present day dreams, by saying that the latter were beyond his control because they were always accompanied by a "short fainting spell." We are therefore justified in saying that there was a direct relationship between the suppressed sexual activities and his fantastic day dreams.

If we bear in mind the different stages described above and follow the act of masturbation we can at once see a distinct analogy. Here as there there is a preliminary craving followed by a pleasurable stage, and the second and third stages of the day dream, the withdrawal from reality and absent mindedness fully correspond to the increasing sexual excitement and its acme at the moment of ejaculation. It is well known that coitus was compared by many writers to a minor epileptic attack. Also the terminal depression corresponds to the same stage of coitus or its inadequate outlet, masturbation. *Post coitum animal triste* is an old saying equally true of masturbation which is always followed by self-reproach.

To illustrate the psychological significance of dreamy states the following case will serve:

Case II.—A., referred to me for treatment by Dr. Frederick Peterson, was a rising journalist of twenty-six years. He was addicted to dreamy states most of which showed the three stages cited above. A few examples recited by himself will give us an idea of their nature: "I am running a race and I feel fine because I am sure of winning. I am accidentally struck in the thigh with the spiked shoe of one of my competitors. I am bleeding, but I don't seem to feel it. I am very excited because I am getting ahead of the others. Some trainers try to stop me because they imagine I am hurt, but I punch them and run on. I win the race, but collapse from exhaustion. I am carried out amidst the applause of the crowd."

"I am taking a walk with a party of young men and women. We are held up by a highwayman. We all submit to it. I stand with my hands up, but taking advantage of the highwayman's momentary inattention I throw myself upon him, take away his pistol and strike him on the head with it. I beat him into submission and then lead him by the collar to the police station amidst the great applause of my companions, who, being Jews, are astonished at my bravery.

"I escape from home and make my way to China. I insinuate myself into court and become a favorite of the Dowager Empress. I am put in charge of the army which I train to great efficiency. A rebellion breaks out. I lead the army. The emperor, who is on the other side is killed or dies (vague). As a reward for my services I marry the Dowager Empress who looks like my mother. This happiness does not last very long, for I am deposed and returned to New York an exile."

The patient stated that these day dreams usually came when he was writing and that they were entirely beyond his control. He himself referred to them "as a sort of absent-mindedness during which I am like a somnambulist."

It is interesting to note that in both patients the dreams appeared during mental concentration. This fully corroborates what Freud states in his Three Contributions to the Sexual Theory, viz., that mental application to an intellectual accomplishment will often result, especially in youthful persons, in a simultaneous sexual excitement. Another striking point in all these dreamy states is the emotional lability in the different stages. The dreamer distinctly realizes that the first two stages are of a pleasurable nature, while the last stage is of a depressive painful nature.

I shall not go into long analytical explanations. I will content myself by stating that here, too, the day dreams were substitutes for the abandoned masturbation and will proceed with the analysis of day dreams proper.

We have said above that the psychosexual constitution of the individual is made up of many components and partial impulses which run through a definite evolution. These impulses are active in infancy, but normally they are gradually repressed, leaving only slight traces of their former existence. As we discussed this question above I shall briefly refer to the impulses of exhibitionism and cruelty only.

It is well known that unlike adults, children like to show themselves naked, that is they like to exhibit. It is not at all unusual to see children of both sexes exposing themselves *coram publico.* Shame is a matter of training. I know a little girl of six years, who at the age of three or four used to invite her grown-up acquaintances to be present while she took her bath and who now blushes at any allusion to it. That the Golden Rule is not inherent in the human being is also well known. Cruelty in our sense is common to childhood. I believe it is La Fontaine who calls childhood "an age without pity." That cruelty and exhibitionism are intimately connected with sex is hardly necessary to mention. Naturalists and anthropologists have repeatedly called attention to it. Freud, who has perhaps penetrated deeper then any one else, shows[10] that when these inpulses are repressed by a process of training and education they form certain reactions like modesty and sympathy which go to make up the character of the individual. But as no impulse is entirely suspended, one can always find some traces of it in the individual's character. Thus persons inclined to obscene joking usually conceal a desire to exhibit and persons having a strong sadistic or cruel component in their sexuality, which is more or less inhibited, are most successful with the tendency wit of aggression.[11] If for some reason these impulses cannot be repressed or when later in life there is a failure of repression, the individual remains a sexual exhibitionist or sadist, or he suffers from a neurosis in which these impulses come to the surface in some negative form. One of the distressing symptoms for which A. sought relief was an irresistible impulse to pinch women. His fancies simply reflected his symptoms. The first two day dreams nicely illustrate, in a rather hidden form, his exhibitionism as well as his sadism. The third one, referring to his marrying the dowager empress who looked like his mother, shows a very nice unconscious mechanism, the so-called Oedipus complex.[12] His neurosis is the result of a conflict between his conscious resistances and his unconscious attachment to his mother. As with every little boy, his mother was the first woman he loved, but unlike the others his libido remained fixed on her. This is a very common mechanism and, as shown by Abraham, accounts for so many consanguineous marriages. Neurotics, who are unconsciously attached to their parents, either never marry because "no girl is like mother" or marry some member of the family who resembles the parent. As a little boy our patient often found home too small for him and his father. He was his rival, as it were, for his mother's affection and for that reason he often wished him dead. Now as a grown-up man he still finds life burdensome because he cannot tolerate his superiors who take the place of his father and he consequently entertains murderous thoughts toward them. The morning before this day dream he read about the war in China and that the army had been trained by foreign officers. This was the main determinant of the last dream, but the other elements that enter into its formation are part and parcel of his neurosis. In his day dreams he runs away from home and becomes a great man, because in reality he dislikes the idea of having to stay at home and be supported by his parents who lately referred to it rather unkindly. In this rebellion he either kills the emperor or he dies. Such vague statements occurring in day or night dreams indicate a marked repression. Here the emperor stands for his father.[13] He thus kills his father and is united to his childhood ideal. But, as he is no longer a child, the dream shows the influence of the incest barriers which were formed during his development. He is therefore deposed and returned to New York an exile. This sudden fiasco is also constellated by the depressive emotional tone of the terminal stage of masturbation which invests, so to say, the last stage of the day dream and determines its character. That A.'s first two day dreams lack the depressive thoughts which go to make up the terminal stage of masturbation is not without reason.

I have purposely selected these examples because they demonstrate a rather interesting mechanism. They always appeared after the patient practised interrupted masturbation. As you know this is a common practice of masturbators, who imagine that loss of seminal fluid is loss of vitality.

In conclusion it may be said that this type of day dreaming is simply a substitution for the abandoned masturbation. The unrequited libido seeking an outlet invests those thoughts which are in some way connected with the individual's hopes and strivings. Like the wolf in the lamb's skin they look quite innocent at first sight, but on closer investigation it becomes very evident that they represent repressed wishes of the person's psychosexual life and thus constitute a concealed form of mental masturbation.

References

1. Freud: Selected Papers on Hysteria, p. 195.

2. For the Mechanism of Identification, see Chap. VI.

3. Freud: Allgemeines über den hysterischen Anfall, Sammlung kleiner Schriften zur Neurosenlehre, Second series, Deuticke, Wien.

4. Zentralblatt für Nervenheilkunde, August, 1909.

5. Ueber hysterische Traumzustände, Jahrbuch für Psychoanalyse Vol. II.

6. *Cf.* Chap. III.

7. *L. c.*

8. *Cf.* Chap. II.

9. *L. c.*

10. Three contributions to the Sexual Theory, translated by A. A. Brill.

11. *Cf.* Chap. XII.

12. *Cf.* Chap. IX.

13. This is a rather common identification, see Freud: The Interpretation of Dreams; also Chap. IX.

CHAPTER IX

THE OEDIPUS COMPLEX

The latent influence on normal persons; its negative manifestations in the psychoneuroses and psychoses

Of the many interesting and valuable discoveries furnished to us through psychanalysis none is as important as those facts which treat of the individual's relation to the family and society. In our psychanalytic work with patients we find that parents play the leading part in their infantile psychic life. This fact is so universal and important that we may say that unless it is thoroughly elaborated and discussed with the patient no analysis is complete or effective. Studies made on psychoneurotics amply demonstrate that contrary to the accepted opinions neurotics are only exaggerations of the normal and that the modes of reaction in both are about the same. The only difference lies in the fact that one can adjust himself to his environments while the other finds it difficult or impossible to do so. If one should ask wherein these difficulties lie the experienced psychanalyst would readily point to the parents. Indeed the more we study the psychoneuroses and the psychoses the clearer it becomes that the most potent factor in their determination is the early parental influence. That our parents should play a leading part in our lives is so obvious that it hardly needs further dilatation. The strange part of it, however, is the fact that these relations are not as amicable or peaceful as seems at first sight. What I mean to say is that, contrary to general belief, there is usually not much love lost between parents and children and that especially little children do not always love their parents in a manner generally accepted. On the contrary they show a marked dislike for one of their parents. This statement may sound very bold and unfounded, but if you will stop to think for a moment you will soon feel that it contains a familiar note. Observation teaches that our love for parents is not innate and spontaneous and that it follows the same laws as that among strangers. Although Freud gave us the true psychological explanation of this conception the principle of it must have keen known from time immemorial. History and every-day life demonstrate it. We all know the fifth commandment: Honor thy father and thy mother, that thy days may be long in the land which the Lord thy God giveth thee. Here we have a direct order to honor our parents and judging by the other commandments and by our modern laws, it must be concluded that to neglect parents was just as natural in the Biblical times as were those impulses against which commandments beginning with "Thou shalt not" had to be imposed. For it is a fact that there is no necessity of commanding the individual to realize his impulses. Left to himself he would constantly try to realize them, and civilization, so called, simply consists of inhibitions imposed upon the individual by religion and society. The more one can inhibit his primitive impulses the more cultured he is, and savages and children must be taught inhibition to fit them for society. To cite Freud: "A progressive renouncement of constitutional impulses, the activity of which afford the ego primary pleasure, seems to be one of the basic principles of human culture."[1]

When we enter into the deeper mental mechanisms of our patients and investigate their love lives, we usually find that the little boy is more attached to his mother and the little girl to her father. In other words, the first woman a boy loves is his mother. The little boy therefore finds his father in the way—he is his rival. When the father is not at home the little son has no one with whom to share his mother's affection. He is therefore angry and jealous of his father and often wishes him dead. One of my patients vividly recalls that at the age of four years he asked his mother whom she loved best him or his father, and when she said that she loved his father best he became furious and cried for hours. Such primitive feelings help to make up the fateful sum of material furnished by the psychic impulse which is formed during the infantile period and which is of great importance for the symptoms appearing in the later neurosis. I could trace directly the symptoms of the cases that I have analyzed to such mechanisms. In normal persons we find the traces of this early love in the dreams of the death of near relatives especially the father.[2]

The sexual feeling for the mother and jealousy of the father is called by Freud the Oedipus complex because antiquity has furnished us with legendary material to confirm this fact. To put it in his words: "The deep and universal effectiveness of these legends can only be explained by granting a similar universal applicability to the above-mentioned assumption in infantile psychology."[3]

The legend referred to is the drama King Oedipus by Sophocles. Laius, the king of Thebes, married Jocasta. After years of childless marriage Laius visited the Delphian Apollo and prayed for a child. The answer of the god was as follows: "Your prayer has been heard and a son will be given to you, but you will die at his hand for Zeus decided to fulfil the curse of Pelops whose son you have once kidnapped." In spite of the warning the son was born, but soon thereafter the child's feet were pierced and tied, and he was delivered to a faithful servant to be exposed in the desert. The servant, however, gave the child to a Corinthian shepherd who took it to his master, King Polybus, who, being childless, adopted it and called it Oedipus, meaning swollen feet. When the boy grew up into manhood he became uncertain of his own origin and consulting the oracle received the following answer: "Beware that thou shouldst not murder thy father and marry thy mother." In order to avoid the fulfilment of this prophecy Oedipus at once left Corinth and accidentally wandered toward Thebes. On the way he met King Laius and struck him dead in a sudden quarrel. He then came to the gates of Thebes where he solved the riddle of the Sphinx who barred his way. As a reward for this he was elected king and presented with the hand of Jocasta. He reigned in peace for many years and begot two sons and two daughters upon his unknown mother until a plague broke out which caused the Thebans to consult the oracle. The messengers returned with the advice that the plague would stop as soon as the murderer of King Laius would be driven from the country. Sophocles then develops the play in a psychanalytic manner until the true relations are discovered, namely, that Oedipus killed his father and married his own mother. The drama ends by Oedipus blinding himself and wandering away into voluntary exile.

In his characteristic penetrating way Freud draws many interesting conclusions some of which I shall mention. Oedipus Tyrannus is a tragedy of fate. Its tragic effect is said to be found in the opposition between the powerful will of the gods and the futile resistance of the human being who is threatened with destruction. The tragedy teaches resignation to the will of God and confession of one's own helplessness. This tragedy has lately been revived by Max Rheinhard and had a long and successful run in Berlin and London. From what we have read, it would seem that it moves modern men no less than it moved the contemporary Greek. In our own times one occasionally witnesses a play dealing with the incest problem which is as tremenduously effective as the Greek drama. I can recall only one such play, The City, by Clyde Fitch. This seems to indicate that the explanation of this fact cannot lie merely in the assumption that the effect of the Greek tragedy is based upon the opposition between human fate and human will, but is to be sought in the peculiar nature of the material by which the opposition is shown. There must be something in us which is prepared to recognize the compelling power of fate in Oedipus while we justly condemn the situations occurring in tragedies of later date as arbitrary inventions. Witness, *e.g.*, the storm that has been produced in this country by Synge's Irish play "The

Play-boy of the Western World," which is a veiled Oedipus complex. Freud states that there must be a factor corresponding to this inner voice in the story of king Oedipus. "His fate moves us only for the reason that it might have been ours, for the oracle has put the same curse upon us before our birth as upon him. Perhaps we are all destined to direct our first sexual impulses toward our mothers and our first hatred and violent wishes toward our father. Our dreams convince us of it. King Oedipus who killed his father and married his mother, is nothing but the realized wish of our childhood. But more fortunate than he we have since succeeded, unless we have become psychoneurotics, in withdrawing our sexual impulses from our mothers and in forgetting our jealousy of our fathers. We recoil from the person for whom this primitive wish has been fulfilled with all the force of the repression which these wishes have suffered within us. By his analysis showing us the guilt of Oedipus the poet urges us to recognize our own inner self, in which these impulses, even if suppressed, are still present."[4]

That the Oedipus legend originated in an extremely old dream material which consists of the painful disturbance of the relation toward one's own parents by means of the first impulses of sexuality, is unmistakably shown in the very text of Sophocles. Jocasta, comforting Oedipus, mentions to him the dream which is dreamed by so many people: "For it has already been the lot of many men in dreams to think themselves partners of their mother's bed. But he passes most easily through life to whom those circumstances are trifles."[5] The dream of having sexual intercourse with one's own mother occurred at that time as it does to-day to many persons who tell it with indignation and astonishment. As may be understood it is the key to the tragedy and the compliment to the dream of the death of the father. The story of Oedipus is the reaction of the imagination to these two typical dreams and, just as the dream when occurring to an adult is experienced with feelings of resistance, so the legend must contain terror and self chastisement. An uncomprehending secondary elaboration tries to make it serve theological purposes.

From my own experience I can fully corroborate Freud's claims. I have on record thirty-eight dreams of sexual relation with one's own mother given to me by twenty-one patients. These dreams were quite plain and there was very little distortion to them. About half of these dreamers reported these dreams before they ever heard of any Oedipus complex, while the other half told about them after I had explained the mechanism. They all assured me that they were perfectly aware of these dreams and to my question why they had not told me before they invariably answered that it was too terrible and revolting a thing to tell, and that the only reason why they told them to me was because they were happy to know they were not the only ones having such dreams. I can say the same of nineteen women who dreamed that they had sexual relations with their fathers. I analyzed Oedipus dreams in which only the father or the mother was masked. Thus one of my female homosexuals told me that the only erotic dreams in which a man played a part was one of having had sexual intercourse with one of our Governors, but on associating to the dream, she told me that she was accustomed to refer to her father as the governor. As you know the president, governor and mayor in dreams usually means the father.[6]

Most of the Oedipus dreams, however, usually show a symbolization of the sexual act in which the parents may be quite plain. One of my patients dreamed that he climbed up a high water tower on a revolving staircase. On reaching midway he met his mother, who accompanied him to the top. The climbing became more and more difficult. He had to hold on very tightly to her for fear that they would both fall. They finally reached the top in a very exhausted state where they both laid down in bed together for a long rest. This patient slept with his mother until he was eighteen years old and, from his own admission, although he entertained no conscious sexual feelings toward her, he wished on at least a few occasions that he could marry her. To those acquainted with dream analysis this dream needs no further elucidation.[7]

A man of thirty-five years reported to me the following dream: "*I dreamt that I was in bed with my mother and as she was talking aloud I told her to be quiet as I was afraid that my father who was in the next room would hear us.*"

This patient was treated for psychosexual impotence and this dream came after unsuccessfully attempting heterosexual intercourse. He was his mother's favorite and owing to the fact that his father was a psychopathic individual who abused and terrified his family he hated him and was much attached to his mother. Whenever his father went on a rampage his mother would lock herself in a room with him, and they often lived through in reality the experience described in the dream. This was also the reason for his sleeping with his mother up to the age of ten years. Disappointed in her husband she lavished all her affection on her son who supplied her with the love she craved. The patient stated that for years he was subject to nightmares showing almost the same content as the above-mentioned dream.

To understand the full significance of this dream it will be necessary to review a few psychological facts.

As stated above we are all destined to direct our first sexual impulses to our mothers. The first woman loved is one's own mother. It is the mother who impresses on the mind the woman-image which remains as a permanent standard for the female ideal. Normally a repression takes place and the boy gradually projects his love to strangers. Investigation shows that the love life of an individual begins at a very early age and as this progresses the love for one's mother gradually fades from consciousness. In the unconscious it remains forever and acts as a constant guide in the future selection of a woman.[8] Every woman in compared to the mother-image and *cœteris paribus*, the closer the resemblance the stronger the woman attracts us. This may shade from the normal to the abnormal. As examples I can cite the following cases:

A very cultured man was attracted only by very stout servants. No other type of woman appealed to him Analysis showed that his first sexual impulses were aroused by a servant girl of that type who took the place of his mother.

A refined married woman of twenty-four years suffered from psychosexual frigidity, but was sexually excited whenever she saw a lame man. This was due to an identification with her mother who had an illicit love affair with a man when she was three or four years old. Like a great many grown-ups her mother considered her little girl an unthinking being and took no pains to conceal anything from her. When her paramour sustained a fracture of his leg and she found it necessary to make frequent calls on him she took her little daughter with her so as to avoid gossip. Although what she witnessed apparently made no impression on her at the time it nevertheless acted as a sexual trauma and formed an association between sex and lameness.[9] This was also determined by the fact that at a later age this lame man took the place of her own father by marrying her widowed mother.

A young married woman who is dominated by a veritable prostitution complex carried on illicit relations with men while she lived with her husband. Psychanalysis showed that she was an only daughter and although her father's pet she saw very little of him during her early childhood as his affairs took him away from home. As far as her memory reached she recalled witnessing unholy loves between her mother and "strange men." She herself married a man who not only belongs to the same type as her father, but who even follows her father's vocation. She thus identified herself with her mother in every respect.

I could quote many more cases,[10] but these will suffice to show the unconscious parental influence. Such influences are found in every person and although they are usually quite harmless they sometimes act perniciously.

This is particularly true of only or favorite children who are overburdened with love. They are not allowed to follow the different stages of the psychosexual evolution and their libido remains fixed on the mother.[11] The result of such a process may be psychosexual impotence. By preventing the boy from projecting his love to strangers there results an unconscious incestuous fixation on the mother which then acts as an inhibition to sexual relations with other women.[12]

Let us return to the above-mentioned dream. From what we know of dreams we may say that those which are accompanied by fear are of a sexual nature. The fear is the converted libido and takes the place of the distortion usually found in other dreams. In other words the dream represents a repressed wish to sleep with his mother and the converted libido is masked behind the fear for the father. His father was furious whenever he found him sleeping with his mother and our patient dreaded lest he should be detected by his father. The dream repeats the same state of mind and thus gives us the key to his neurosis. By sleeping with his mother to so late an age the incestuous feelings were kept alive and fixed on her, but as he grew older he energetically defended himself against them and finally succeeded in repressing them from consciousness. As a reaction to these unconscious desires he became extremely moral and religious and avoided anything sexual. At the age of twenty-eight he attempted coitus for the first time and failed. This failure was repeated at every subsequent attempt. He could not accomplish the sexual act because of the sexual fixation on the mother. Every woman unconsciously recalled his mother and, because of the marked repression coitus was naturally impossible. This was also constellated by his unconscious fear of his father. The patient was cured of his impotence as soon as these mechanisms were laid bare and explained to him.

Conscious incestuous feelings and experiences in adult life are not as rare as one would imagine. This subject has been discussed by Krafft-Ebing, Bloch, Havelock Ellis and others. My own observations in this regard taught me that sexual feelings and fancies about one's parents, sisters and brothers are not only extremely common in early life, but that they also exist later. Nor must it be imagined that whenever it is found we deal with defective persons. The individual circumstances must always be considered. Havelock Ellis[13] explains the abhorence of incest on the basis of familiarity. He states that "The normal failure of the pairing instinct to manifest itself in the case of brothers and sisters or of boys and girls brought up together from infancy is a merely negative phenomenon due to the inevitable absence under those circumstances of the conditions which evoke the pairing impulse" (p. 205). "Passion between brothers and sisters is, indeed, by no means so rare as is sometimes supposed, and it may be very strong, but it is usually aroused by the aid of those conditions which are normally required for the appearance of passion, more especially by the unfamiliarity caused by long separation" (p. 206). I agree with Havelock Ellis as far as he goes, but it seems to me that unfamiliarity plays only a subordinate part in the promotion of certain feelings between brothers and sisters. Unfamiliarity does not necessarily cause attraction between strangers of the opposite sexes, but long separation, especially when occurring since early life, is sure to produce a strong fascination between brothers and sisters. This is due to the repressed Oedipus complex. As was said above, every woman that later comes into the individual's life is unconsciously compared to the mother image in our unconscious. It is quite obvious that the sister fits into this image much better than any other woman. Who resembles the mother more than the daughter? Besides, the daughter has the advantage over the mother of youth and beauty. In this connection I would like to give an incident related to me by a colleague:

He came to this country from Germany at the age of fourteen years having left at home a sister one and a half years his junior. Years later he visited an exhibition in the Grand Central Palace in New York City and was strongly fascinated by a young lady he saw there. The attraction was so strong that he lost interest in the exhibits and followed her around until she left the place. Nor did this fascination end here. He told me that for months he acted like a man in love and for years he measured every woman by his "Grand Central Girl." He returned to his native city after having been eighteen years in America and as soon as he saw his younger sister the thought flashed through his mind, "Here is my Grand Central Girl." There was, indeed, a remarkable resemblance between his sister and the unknown young woman with whom he fell in love in America. His sister was the picture of his mother.

Moreover in real life, daughters often take the place of

their mothers. I know of a few cases where men first loved the mothers and then switched over to the daughters. The daily press sometimes reports such cases.[14]

It is in the psychoses, however, that one sees the marked influence of the Oedipus complex. Here the complex usually comes to the surface in the form of symptoms, usually hallucinations and delusions, and the analysis can generally trace these automatisms to early repressed feelings and experiences. The following cases will serve as paradigms:

CASE I.—V, twenty-nine years old, suffers from the paranoid form of dementia præcox. He hears voices accusing him of having had sexual relations with his mother. Analysis showed that as a boy he entertained sexual fancies about his mother. He often looked through the keyhole when she took her bath.

CASE II.—Mrs. F., a married woman of twenty-eight years, is a paranoid præcox. For more than a year she has been laughing and talking to herself uttering words like "clean, never, respectable, not at all, none." When questioned she states that she hears voices who accuse her of having been "too intimate with her father and brother" and the words uttered are only answers to her imaginary accusers. They read as follows: I am clean. I never did such terrible things. I am respectable. It is not at all true that I had sexual relations with my father and brother."

CASE III.—With Dr. H. Valentine Wildman I have recently committed a young man to the River Crest Sanatorium. This patient was paranoid and his main delusions were fairly well systematized. They were directed against his mother. He called her vile names and accused her of having made sexual advances to him. The following remarks pointing to a retrospective falsification contain the nucleus of his delusions: "I remember when I was a kid, she (mother) looked at my eyes and then paced the floor as if to say 'you are for me' and since then she wanted to make me her lover." The history of the case shows the typical mechanisms of paranoia, that is, there was fixation in narcism and mother love (he was the mother's favorite),

defence against homosexual wish phantasies, then failure of repression, as manifested in some homosexual experiences and delusions of persecution.[15]

Now it may be asked whether children show by their behavior any indication of the Oedipus complex and whether fathers realize consciously that their sons are their rivals. Anamneses taken from normal and abnormal persons answer these questions in the affirmative. Also the works of Freud, Bleuler, Jung, Putnam, Ferenczi, Stekel, Abraham, Rank, Jones,[16] and others, show beyond any doubt that this is the case. To quote Bleuler, "After our attention had been called to it we found this Oedipus complex more and more frequently. It is also an important factor in the selection of lovers among normal and abnormal persons."[17] I have collected many, many facts. Some I have personally observed and some were given to me by reliable colleagues and friends, showing that beyond any doubt small children often wish to replace the parent of their own sex. A brilliant little boy of three years, hearing that he will sleep with his mother because his father was going to stay away for the night, expressed his great pleasure to his mother and added "Let us play that we are married. I'll call you Mary and you call me John" (names of parents). Later when he entered his mother's sleeping room he said "Here comes your husband." A little girl of three and one-half years on being punished by her mother exclaimed in her childish way, "Go away to Susie (her dead sister), I can be papa's Mama (meaning his wife, as her father calls her mother 'mama')." Another little girl of about four years kissed her father and kept on repeating "I love you so much, papa. Let's go to the

Bronx and never come home to mama." And on being questioned she admitted that she did not love her mother.

It is not uncommon for parents to be jealous of the love shown by the other parent for the child. A glaring example of this kind was reported to me by a patient referred to me by Dr. Coriat of Boston. Her husband was a very prominent business man, but somewhat psychopathic. She was very much attached to her only son and the more she loved him the more he was hated by the father. The latter openly expressed his jealousy and hatred for his son and treated him most cruelly whenever he could do so. This feeling continued for more than thirty years until the father died, and was the cause of much unhappiness.

In his study on incest among savages[18] Freud showed that the incest shyness is an infantile trait and in striking accord with the psychic life of the neurotic. Psychanalysis teaches that the first sexual object of the boy is of an incestuous prohibitive nature directed against the mother or sister; it also shows us how the developing individual frees himself from these feelings. The neurotic individual, however, regularly represents a fragment of psychic infantilism. He is either unable to free himself from the infantile relations of psychosexuality, or he returned to them. It is for that reason that the incestuous fixations of the libido continue to play a great part in his unconscious psychic life.

References

1. Sammlung kleine Schriften zur Neurosenlehre, Zweite Fogel.
2. Freud: The Interpretation of Dreams. The Macmillan Co.

New York, and George Allen Co., London.

3. Freud: *L. c.*, p. 221.

4. *L. c.*, p. 223.

5. Act IV, Sc. 3, translated by Clark.

6. Freud: *L. c.* p. 246

7. Freud: *L. c.* p. 246. On Stairway Dreams.

8. *Cf.* Chap. X.

9. For the mechanism of such traumas see Freud: Selected papers on Hysteria, p. 159.

10. Most of the cases described by Mantegazza as Idiogamists probably belong to this category: Zeitschrift f. Sexualwissenschaft, p. 223.

11. *Cf.* Chap. X.

12. Ferenzi: Analytische Deutung und Behandlung der psychosexuellen Impotenz beim Manne. Psychiatrisch-neurologische Wochenschrift, 1908, No. 35. See also the works of Stekel and Steiner.

13. Sexual Selection in Man, p. 204.

14. Those who are interested in the problem may read an excellent paper on the subject by Freud: Die Inzestscheu der Wilden; Imago, Heft 1.

15. For full particulars of these mechanisms, see Chap. VI.

16. See especially, "The Oedipus Complex as an explanation of Hamlet's Mystery, Amer. Jour. of Psychology, Jan., 1910.

17. Dementia Præcox oder Gruppe der Schizophrenien, p. 344. Deuticke, Leipzig u. Wien, 1911.

18. Freud: *L. c.*

CHAPTER X

THE ONLY OR FAVORITE CHILD IN ADULT LIFE

Fixation on early parental images; the psychology of the mother-in-law

Very little attention has been given to the problem of the only child, and the little literature we have at our disposal deals mainly with the superficial and general aspects of the question. Neter, who has written an excellent pamphlet on the subject,[1] gives a very good description of the only child's attributes, but he does not enter into the deeper psychological elements. Moreover, no attempt has been made outside of the Freudian school[2] to follow those children into adult life and to trace the individual influence at play in their adjustment to environments. This can be readily understood when we remember that very little has been done in child psychology in general and that only few psychologists are at present occupying themselves with the subject.

Stimulated by the works of Freud[3] and Jung[4] I have investigated the subject from the psychanalytical side and shall endeavor to present some of the results. But before proceeding to do so it will be necessary to orient ourselves on some of the psychological principles that form a part of the discussion.

In his famous essay *Concerning Human Understanding,* Locke tells us that the child's mind is essentially a *tabula rasa,* a tablet upon which nothing is written, and that all knowledge rests on experience. Psychanalysis fully demonstrates Lock's empiricism, and confining ourselves to the question of parental influences and relationships we may say that every individual's mind possesses certain stereotype plates or models, as it were, which are the result of mental impressions produced by the parents during childhood. Thus a father image[5] and a mother image remain permanently engraved in the mind and act as standards for estimation of men and women that later enter into this person's life. It is not difficult to show that our behavior toward our fellow beings depends mostly on our relations to our parents. In other words we unconsciously endeavor to fit every stranger into one of our latent parental images and our likes and dislikes depend in a great measure on the success or failure of such correlation. Further investigation shows that children do not always love their parents as is commonly supposed, but very often hate one of them. The first woman the little boy loves is her mother, and the first man the little girl loves is her father. The little boy idolizes his mother and supplies her with that part of poetic love which she no longer gets from her husband. The mother calls her little boy sweetheart and tries to realize in him her ideal of the man. The same thing takes place between the little girl and her father. Normally, however, these parental ideals vanish with the advancing age, when the growing child begins to project his love on strangers. The boy then no longer thinks that his mother is the prettiest and loveliest woman in the world, but he evinces an interest in other persons of the opposite sex. The deflection of love from the mother may also be furthered by the appearance of a little brother, who claims a part of his mother's love and attention. However, this absence of the mother ideal is only apparent. It is not eliminated, but repressed into the unconscious and there it continues to exert its influence throughout the whole life of the individual. Psychanalysis of normal persons shows beyond any doubt the enormous influence of unconscious parental complexes. It explains the important mechanism of transference[6] as well as many of the peculiarities of the love life.[7]

Recently I was consulted by a young girl of twenty-one years who was said to have become nervous as a result of a disagreement with her mother. She was in love with a man of forty-six years to whom her mother strongly objected, not only on account of the marked difference in their ages, but because the man was considered mentally abnormal. During our conversation she remarked that her mother had always been in her way and by way of explanation she stated that her mother was jealous of her and that when she was younger she hated to have her mother go along when she went out with her father. "I always looked upon her as a stranger," she said. She idolized her father who is her ideal in every respect, although he is a paranoiac and has been for years in an insane asylum. She surprised me when she told me that there is as marked a difference in the ages of her father and mother as there is in her own and her fiancé's ages. Indeed, all the features of the case unmistakably pointed to an identification with her mother and an unconscious desire to get her father ideal. Such cases are not at all uncommon; I have given some in the preceding chapter and could cite many more.

From what has just been said it can be readily understood that such parental influences may often be strong enough to inhibit materially the individual's relations to the other sex. Thus, too much and prolonged affection on the part of the mother is apt to cause an undue conscious or unconscious attachment to the parents, and thus prevent the child from going through the various stages of its psychosexual development. We know that the sexual impulse of childhood is autoerotic or objectless.[8] The child knows no other sexual object than himself and gets his gratification through the erogenous zones of his own body. As it grows older we have the so-called latency period, during which the greater part of the sexual excitation is utilized for aims other than sexual, viz., for the formation of social feelings and the future sexual barriers. Between autoerotism and the object love there is an intermediate stage which has been designated as narcism. Freud tells us that every stage of development of the psychosexual life offers a possibility for "fixation" which may result in a type of character. Thus we know that fixation in narcism may cause paranoia[9] or homosexuality, and that fixation in autoerotism may lay the foundation for dementia præcox. By giving the child too much love, mothers often prolong or cause a fixation in the various stages mentioned. This naturally occurs very often in only children, who, having no one with whom to share their parents' affection, are overburdened with love. The same takes place in favorite children who are subjected to the same conditions as only children durıng the impressionable period of their existence. Since the fall of 1908 I have examined 400 only or favorite children, and my findings may be divided into (*a*) general and (*b*) specific.

(*a*) Whether *burdened by heredity or not* the adult only child usually shows one prominent feature, namely, he is a very poor competitor in the struggle for existence. Having been carefully reared and constantly watched by his loving mother, he remains forever "mama's boy." He is devoid of those qualities which characterize the real boy. He lacks independence, self-confidence and the practical skill which the average boy acquires through competition with other boys.

Owing to the fact that the only boy constantly associates with grown-ups he is usually precocious even in childhood, and as he grows older he finds it very hard to associate with persons of his own age. I know an only boy of nineteen years who has not a single friend. He is practically asocial. He wishes only to associate with persons much older than himself and cannot adapt himself to the society of young people because they "bore" him. Some time ago I was consulted about another only boy, seven years old, because, as his mother put it, he did not get along with other children and was real blase. He was not interested in anything. Toys, pets, books, etc., that would have been sufficient to delight the hearts of a dozen children had absolutely no charm for him. He was in constant need of new excitements and as they could not be supplied quickly enough he was unhappy and morose.

The only child is usually spoiled and coddled because the parents gratify all his whims and have not the heart to be severe with or punish him when necessary. This has its evil consequences in adult life, for the slightest depreciation, hardly noticeable by the average person, is enough to throw him into a fit of depression and rage lasting for days and even for weeks. An only daughter attempted suicide because her best friend received more attention than she at a social gathering.

It is due to the undivided attention and abnormal love that the only child gets from his parents that he develops into a confirmed egotist. He is never neglected in favor of sisters and brothers. He is the sole ruler of the household and his praises are constantly sung. It is, therefore, no wonder that the only child becomes vain and one-sided and develops an exaggerated opinion of himself. In later life he is extremely conceited, jealous and envious. He begrudges the happiness of friends and acquaintances and he is therefore shunned and disliked.* A favorite son, a bachelor of sixty-two years who was a wealthy retired merchant, told me that whenever there was a rise in the market he suffered from severe depression and fits of envy, simply because he knew that some of his friends would make money. He himself had no personal interest in the market. Such qualities are surely not conducive to happiness, and it is not at all surprising that almost all such children are selfish, unhappy and morose.

(*b*) The specific findings are of still greater interest. Of the 400 cases observed there were 172 men and 228 women. Their ages ranged from eighteen to sixty-eight years. The morbid manifestations were as follows:

* A typical example is Joseph of the Bible, having been his mother's only son (Rachel died during the birth of Benjamin) and his father's favorite, he was despised and hated by his half-brothers.

The predominant feature in about 36 per cent. of my cases was the abnormal sex life. Most of them sought treatment for homosexuality, psychic impotence (men) and sexual anesthesia (women); there were also some exhibitionists, voyeurs, sadists and masochists. About 18 per cent. suffered from the various types of dementiapræcox. The rest represented the different forms of the psychoneuroses.

No statistical conclusions should be drawn from these figures as most of these patients came or were sent to me for treatment because they suffered from psychoneuroses or from the other maladies enumerated above. They show, however, the marked prevalence of only or favorite children in these classes. Bearing in mind our psychanalytic knowledge of sex this is not at all surprising. The child is born with the germs of sexuality and during the first years of its life is polymorphous perverse. That is, if an adult should manifest any of the sexual activities that we see in the child he would be considered perverse. But as the child grows older most of these perversions undergo repression and the rest are subjugated to the primacy of the genitals which serve the purpose of procreation.[10] It is quite obvious that abnormal love in early life hinders the normal sexual evolution. It either keeps alive or later revives some of the early sexual activities. The boy cannot transfer his libido on other women because his mother stands in his way. As a rule this is accomplished quite innocently under the guise of maternal care. Such mothers discourage social intercourse with the opposite sex because they wish to preserve their son's purity, etc. A number of my homosexual patients told me that their mothers were actually jealous of every woman with whom they chanced to come in contact and behaved exactly as if they were confronted with a rival. No one is good enough for such children. At least that is what the parents think. This, by the way, is one of the secrets of mothers-in-law. They unconsciously want their sons for themselves and are jealous of every other woman. It is a sex jealousy pure and simple.* The majority of only children do not marry at

* The deeper reasons, however, lying at the basis of the hostility between the proverbial mother-in-law and her son-in-law are explained by Freud. (Imago Heft I.) He first shows that among savages the world over there exist very stringent laws against any familiarity with one's mother-in-law. The son-in-law and mother-in-law are forced by the tribal laws to shun each other. They must run away or hide when they meet by chance. In civilized communities where, to the regret of many, there are no such laws, it is extremely common to find very strained, not to say hostile feelings between mother-in-law and son-in-law. Freud uses a term coined by Bleuler to describe the feeling between mother-in-law and son. He thinks that the relation between them may be designated as "ambivalent," *i.e.*, it is made up of both affectionate and hostile feelings. Some of these feelings are quite clear. Thus the mother-in-law dislikes to relinquish her daughter to a stranger whom she suspects, and shows a tendency to assume a domineering attitude which she became accustomed to in her own home. The son-in-law, on the other hand, is determined to resent any subordination to the will of a stranger. He is jealous of all persons who once possessed his wife's love and, what is more, he dislikes to have his illusion of sexual overestimation disturbed. Such disturbance mostly emanates from the mother-in-law who reminds him of his wife because of many common features between them, but who lacks all the attractions of youth, beauty and psychic freshness which give value to his wife.

Added to that there are unconscious motives. Whenever the psychosexual needs of the woman are to be gratified in marriage or in family life she is always threatened by the danger of lack of gratification through a premature cessation of the marital relations or all or they marry some near relative whom they unconsciously identify with their parent image. The *probable average* of my patients' ages was thirty-four years, but only ninety-three out of the 400 had been married. Most of them remained old maids and bachelors.

through the uneventfulness of her emotional life. The ageing mother protects herself against it by living, as it were, in her children. It is said that one remains young with one's children. This is really the most valuable psychic gain accruing to the parents from their children. This living through the daughter proceeds in the mother to an extent that she falls in love with the man her daughter loves, which, in pronounced cases, leads to severe forms of neurotic disturbance brought on by the violent psychic conflicts. A tendency to love her son-in-law is frequently observed in the mother-in-law and either this feeling alone or its contrary emotion allies itself to the tumultuous struggling forces in her psyche. Quite often the son-in-law faces the hostile, sadistic components of the emotions of love which only serve to better repress the prohibited affectionate feelings.

The relations of the man to his mother-in-law are complicated by similar feelings which flow, however, from another source. As a rule the road of object selection leading to the love object is followed by the man over the images of his mother or perhaps his sister. The deflection of his first love from these beloved persons of his childhood is effected by the incest barriers in order that he should attain in a stranger this prototype. In place of his mother or the mother of his sister he is now confronted by the mother-in-law. This gives rise to a tendency to return to the prehistoric selection which is rapidly repressed. His incest shyness demands that he should not be reminded of the geneology of his love selection. The rejection is facilitated by the actuality of the mother-in-law whom he did not know from the beginning of his existence and hence, unlike his mother's, her image does not remain unchanged in his unconscious. A special addition of attractiveness and repulsion to the emotional mixture allows the conjecture that the mother-in-law really represents an incestuous temptation for the son-in-law. On the other hand, it is not rare for a man to fall in love first with his future mother-in-law before turning his affection to her daughter.

With the brief space at my disposal I am unable to enter into any psychological explanation of these different perversions and I must therefore presuppose a knowledge of the Freudian literature on the part of my readers. I merely repeat that parental influences play a great part in both the normal and neurotic individual, but whereas the normal person gets away at least consciously from these dominations the neurotic remains anchored and succeeds only partially in freeing himself from them. This fixation is mainly responsible for psychic impotence, frigidity and homosexuality,[12] and its general influences can always be found in every psychoneurotic.[13] I know an old bachelor of forty-five years, an only son, who slept with his mother until she died four years ago. He is a good business man and is said to be normal in every other respect. I have treated an old maid, a favorite daughter, who lost her father three years ago. She still wears black and cries bitterly at any allusion to her father. She answered as follows my question as to why she still wore mourning: "Why shouldn't I? No one ever had such a kind, generous and self-sacrificing father. There is not another man like him in this world. O! how I love this man, etc." This may sound like pure filial love, but having analyzed her, I have definitely ascertained that she loved her father as any woman loves a stranger. We can readily see why such persons cannot marry. This patient characteristically expressed it when she said: 'If I could find a man like my father I would marry."

Just a few words on prophylaxis. Of course it would be best for the individual as well as the race that there should be no only children. However, when this cannot be avoided by virtue of ill health or death of one of the parents the child need not necessarily become a neurotic and belong to any of the categories mentioned above. It all depends upon its subsequent bringing up.

When we read the history of only children we find that only those who have been brought up wrongly develop into abnormal beings, those who are not pampered and coddled have the same chances as other children. As classical examples we may mention Nero and Confucius, the former was a spoiled only child, while the latter was a well-bred only child. An only child should be made to associate with other children who will soon teach him that he is not the only one in the world. This should begin at a very early age. I have seen many "nervous and wild" only children who were completely changed after a few weeks' attendance in a kindergarten or public school. But what is still more important is that only children should not be gorged with parental love. Parents should take care that such children should not develop an exaggerated idea of their own personality and think that they are superior to everybody. For individuals imbued with such paranoid ideas are bound to come into conflict with their fellow-men. What is true of the individual may also be true of a race, and history furnishes us with a very nice example.

I refer to the only and favorite child of Jehovah, the Jewish race. The Bible tells us that the Jews are the "chosen people," "the only son," and even "the first-born." That the Jews have displayed all the attributes of the only or favorite child need hardly be mentioned. From the Bible we learn that they were stiff-necked, spoiled and overbearing, and considered themselves superior to every other nation. Characteristics of such nature have been attributed to them by almost all writers of ancient and modern times, and although some are gross exaggerations it must nevertheless be admitted that they are essentially correct in reference to the Hebrews of antiquity and the modern orthodox European Jews. Still it is gratifying to note that this no longer holds true of the great bulk of western Jews who have enjoyed a couple of generations of freedom. The explanation of this change is given by Dr. M. Fishberg [14] in his very interesting book. He plainly shows that "Judaism has been preserved throughout the long years of Israel's dispersion by two factors: its separative ritualism, which prevented close and intimate contact with non-Jews, and the iron laws of Christian theocracies of Europe which encouraged and enforced isolation." In other words, as long as the Jew has been imbued with the racial pride of belonging to the "chosen people" and has been offering daily prayers to Jehovah because he was not created a gentile, he perforce remained exclusive and therefore was suspected and disliked by his non-Jewish neighbors. When we study the history of the Jews we find that their enforced isolation was the result of an early, voluntary clannish exclusiveness. This shows the striking analogy to the only boy who at first refuses to associate with others because he believes himself superior to everybody else, and who is later excluded from social relations because he is misunderstood and disliked. Dr. Fishberg also tells us that as soon as the barriers are removed the Jews readily assimilate and all former prejudices disappear. The only boy, too, loses his identity as soon as he realizes that he is no better than his fellow beings.

The problem is more complicated when we come to prophylaxis in relation to psychosexuality and I regret that I am unable to enter here into a long discussion. I shall merely say that parents should remember that proper sex regulation does not necessarily imply repression and extermination of all sex feelings, and that the requisite for perfect manhood and womanhood are all the impulses and desires that are normally common to men and women.

In conclusion I wish to say that the only child is a morbid product of our present social economic system. He is usually an offspring of wealthy parents who, having been themselves brought up in luxury and anxious that their children should share their fate, refuse to have more than one or two children. By their abnormal love they not only unfit the child for life's battle but prevent him from developing into normal manhood, thus producing sexual perverts and neurotics of all descriptions.

References

1. Das einzige Kind. Gmelin, München.

2. A paper was read on this subject by Drs. Sadger and Friedjung before the Vienna Psychoanalytic Society, October 5, 1910.

3. Analyse der Phobie eines 5 jährigen Knaben. Jahrbuch f. Psychoanalyse, Vol. I.

4. Experiences Concerning the Psychic Life of the Child. Translated by A. A. Brill, Am. Jour. of Psychology, April, 1910.

5. Jung: Symbole und Wandlungen der Libido. Jahrbuch f. Psychoanalyse, Vol. II.

6. Freud: Zur Dynamik der Uebertragung. Zentralblatt f. Psychoanalyse, II; and Brill: A Few Remarks on the Technique of Psychanalysis, Medical Review of Reviews, April, 1912.

7. Jung: Die Bedeutung des Vaters für das Schicksal des Einzelnen. Jahrbuch für Psychoanalyse, Vol. I.

8. Three Contributions to the Sexual Theory. Translated by A. A. Brill.

9. *Cf.* Chap. VI.

10. Freud: *L. c.*

11. Abraham: Die Stellung der Verwandtenehe in der Psychologie der Neurosen. Jahrbuch fur Psychoanalyse, Vol. I.

12. Freud: *L. c.*; also Ferenczi: Analytische Deutung der psychosexuellen Impotenz beim Manne. Psychiatr. Neurolog. Wochenschrift, 1908, and the works of Stekel and Sadger.

13. Freud: The Interpretation of Dreams, p. 224.

14. The Jews, A Study of Race and Environment. Scribner's Pub. Co.

CHAPTER XI

ANAL EROTICISM AND CHARACTER

In his Three Contributions to the Sexual Theory Freud shows that the sexual impulse in man consists of many components and partial impulses. Many essential contributions to the sexual excitement are furnished by the peripheral excitement of certain parts of the body, such as the genitals, mouth, anus and bladder outlets which we call erogenous zones. All these zones are active in infancy and only some of them go to make up the sexual life. The others are deflected from the sexual aims and utilized for other purposes. This is the process of sublimation. During the sexual latency period—four to beginning of puberty, eleven—reaction formations like shame, loathing and morality, are formed in the psychic life of the individual at the cost of the excitements furnished by these erogenous zones, which act as dams for the later sexual activity. The anal zone is one of the components of the sexual impulse which, though active in infancy, falls into desuetude in the course of development, for our present cultural life does not use it for sexual purposes. It is the reaction formation of this zone that I shall here discuss.

In the course of psychanalysis we come across patients who tell us that it took them a long time to learn to control their bowels. These patients recall that even in the later years of childhood they occasionally met with an accident. When we investigate still further we find that they belonged to those infants who refused to empty their bowels when placed on the chamber because defecation caused them pleasure. A number of my patients clearly recalled that even in later years they obtained pleasure by withholding their movements, and that they took an unusual interest in their fecal excretions. This usually shows that their sexual constitution brought along an enhanced erogenous significance of the anal zone. As they grew older all these activities disappeared, and instead they manifested a triad of qualities which were described by Freud in his article on Character and Anal Eroticism.[1]

To illustrate this character I shall cite the following case.

X., forty-four years old, divorced, a very successful merchant, was referred to me for treatment by Dr. F. Peterson. The patient stated that his present illness dated back to his twentieth year. On examination it was found that he presented a typical compulsion neurosis,[2] and that some of the compulsive ideas were as follows. When eating soup he would think it urine; when eating sausage he would have to think of feces. The noise of an auto horn made him think of a flatus or horse's flatus, on account of which he gave up automobile riding. On going to sleep he became obsessed by visions of people having movements of the bowels. A woman's mouth made him think of the rectum, her eyes recalled the anus. Shaking hands with a person recalled a man using toilet paper. Looking at big fat persons would obsess him with thoughts of their fecal excrements, the size, consistency, etc. A person with protruding teeth would recall feces protruding from the anus. The moon constantly recalled the rectum.

These are only a few of the many dozens of similar compulsive ideas which forever obsessed him. Besides the obsessions he suffered from chronic constipation and from many other somatic disturbances.

On hearing this voluminous skatological story I naturally thought of the anal eroticism, and the more I became acquainted with my patient the completer the picture became.

Now Freud describes the persons showing the anal eroticism as being especially orderly, economical, and obstinate. Every one of these terms embraces a small group or series of allied characteristic features. Thus orderly includes physical cleanliness as well as scrupulosity in little things; its opposite would be disorder and negligence. Economy may shade into avariciousness; obstinacy may lead to spite and to a tendency for violence and revengeful acts. It is the last two—economy and obstinacy—that hang most firmly together, and are most constantly encountered, though the third is often found in the same person.

X. dressed and looked very neat and gentlemanly. He was very conventional, moved in very nice circles, and tried to make the impression that he was very particular about society matters. Thus he often referred to his friend as not a gentleman because he would not always put on evening dress for theater. The slightest infarction of the general rule offended him. He lived in the best hotels and belonged to some very fine clubs. From his history I found that he was extremely self willed and obstinate. He hated all his brothers because they claimed that he thought he knew it all, and he would give me many instances to show that he really was superior to them. This characteristic was not only apparent in his dealings with his family, but with everyone else including doctors. He consulted physicians in almost every principal city of the U. S. and abroad and spoke disparagingly of all. He had also been a Christian Scientist and a New Thoughter, but as they did not benefit him he put them on the same level with the doctors. It was often very amusing to hear him speak of doctors I knew, and I have no doubt that I fare no better when he talks to others. His obstinacy and revenge led him to enter into commercial competition with his own brothers, and when his older brother implored his help and threatened to blow out his own brains because of financial ruin he not only refused to assist him, but said to him: "Not a cent! Shoot yourself; do you remember how you treated me?" (revenge and spite).

As an illustration of his financial dealings I shall cite an experience I had with him. As I said above he was Dr. Peterson's patient, and I first saw him in Dr. P.'s office. He became unusually friendly, and as soon as an opportunity presented itself he proposed that if I charge him less for the treatment he would leave Dr. P. and come to me. I told him nicely that I could not think of entertaining such a proposition, and that things would have to remain as they were. A few weeks later he saw P. unknown to me, and told him that he was poor and unable to continue with the treatment unless his fees were reduced. Dr. P., not knowing the true circumstances, reduced his fee 50 per cent. That same week he invested many thousands in a new business venture in New York City. More than this, when his bill was sent to him at the end of the month he sent a check for about one-tenth of the amount on account. It is now about two years since the treatment ceased and he still sends us small amounts from time to time. I may here mention that he is a very wealthy man and owns large interests in a number of big commercial houses. His dealings with other people were of a similar nature. Thus, I prescribed some medicine for him and he then complained that the druggist was a highway robber. He lost the friendship of many people because of his stinginess. I have this from his own account. In fine he was what people would call a miser, though to all appearances he looked like a generous gentleman. As a business man he was a great success because, as he said, "I knew how to manage things, and I could always be relied upon."

The extreme neatness, orderliness, and reliability in our patient are nothing but reaction formations against the interest in the not neat or dirty which is not a part of the body.

During the analysis I found that as a child the patient had a hard time to control his rectum. He was punished and jeered for regularly soiling himself up to his sixth year. At nine years he was sent home from school in disgrace because he broke wind in the class room. This was recalled under marked emotivity. He stated that it was a mixed class of boys and girls which made it still harder to bear. The following year he met with another accident while following a parade. He received a rather severe spanking for it because he had on a new white suit. The patient also recalled that as early as in his fifth year he had the habit of sticking his finger into his rectum, a habit which he continued for years.

Whether he was one of these infants who held back his stools I could not discover, but as far as his memory reached there was an extreme interest for feces and for the gluteal region.

It is not simple to connect the interest in defecation with obstinacy but we must remember that even infants can be self willed when put on the chamber, and that painful irritations of the skin connected with the anal zone (spanking) are utilized to break the child's obstinacy. We all know that when people wish to express spite or spiteful mocking they invite people to kiss their behind, which points to a repressed pleasure. As a child our patient was very often spanked not only by his parents but by his older brother. One incident which he especially remembered was a very brutal treatment by his older brother.

The relation between defecation and money though seemingly remote still shows a definite connection. Some of you know that the most obstinate cases of constipation can be cured by psychanalysis. Of course they can also be cured by other means such as hypnotism, but by psychanalysis they can be cured only after the money complex of the patient has been thoroughly thrashed out and brought to consciousness. We know that misers are called filthy (filthy lucre), and that in mythology, fairy tales, superstitions, and dreams money is intimately connected with feces (goose that laid the golden egg). In the old Babylonian writings gold is the dung of hell.[3] It is also probable that the contrast between the most valuable that man has learned to know and the least valuable which he ejects as refuse has formed the identification. This identification is also strengthened by the fact that when the erotic interest in defecation ceases the interest in money begins which was lacking during childhood. The yellow color which is common to gold and feces probably forms another association.

It may also be mentioned that the triad of qualities are not found in those persons who retain the anus as an erogenous zone; *e.g.,* homosexual pederasts. Those whom I know are all very generous indeed. The treatment of X. had to be stopped on account of his money complex at the end of about two months, although he admitted that he was much benefited by the analysis. When he first came for treatment he was so annoyed by the obsession caused by the noise of auto horns that he promised me 75 per cent. of his income if I rid him of it. After a few weeks' analysis this and some other obsessions were removed, he was very pleased and surprised, he thought it was miraculous, but notwithstanding all this it was impossible for him to pay a moderate fee for his treatment. As far as I have gone the analysis showed an accentuation of the anal zone in infancy, a retarded repression with its reaction formation, as shown by his character, and then a failure of the repression at the age of 20 years with a negative revival of the anal activity in the form of the skatological obsessions.

Case II.—T., thirty years old, suffered for years from a compulsion neurosis which manifested itself in obsessions, doubts, and phobias. To save time I shall merely state that he soiled himself to the age of three years, and from his mother's account he was almost never free from bowel trouble until the age of five years. The neurosis manifested itself at fifteen years, and besides many obsessive thoughts he was also troubled by an obsessive act. He could not resist the impulse to rub his feces on walls, and at times on his body. T. stated that he had the habit of holding back his bowels because it gave him a distinct feeling of pleasure and stimulated his mental activity. Whenever he was confronted with a difficult task he "practised constipation." As an example he gave the following episode. As a reporter for a newspaper he was sent to observe and report the manœuvres of the National Guard. He was very anxious to write nice reports and to accomplish this he would hold back his movements for two to three days until it became almost unbearable, and he would then imagine himself on the battle field of Waterloo and describe what he saw. Here, too, the anal activities were the result of a failure in the repression of an enhanced zone.

But it often happens that in addition to an erogenous zone there is also a revival of one or more of the partial impulses. Whenever this occurs the symptoms usually show a corresponding combination. The following will serve as an illustration.

Case III.—B., thirty-nine years old, suffered from a compulsion neurosis. He was obsessed with doubts and phobias which referred to definite ideas about people being killed. It would be impossible to give here a description of this very interesting case which I hope to report in full at some future date. I simply wish to state that he too, showed an enhanced anal activity in infantile life, although no nearly as marked as in the other cases. But the most prominent factor in his infantile sexuality was the component of cruelty. B. was taught to use firearms at a very early age. His greatest pleasure up to the age of nine to ten years was shooting birds, squirrels and rabbits. At the age of puberty he became very sympathetic, and one day after shooting a squirrel he suddenly experienced feelings of compassion and remorse. Since then he found it very hard to go out shooting. When his neurosis developed at the age of eighteen years he also began to suffer from constipation which continued ever since for fifteen years. No medication would relieve him until he accidentally discovered that the following process gave him a movement of the bowels. He once played with a spool of cotton upon which was a picture of a child. He rolled it and when the child's picture came his way he stuck a pin into it. After five minutes of such play he would have a movement. He then resorted to this practice which he modified from time to time until he was cured. He carried a number of long pins which he sharpened from time to time, and every morning he drew a picture of a girl and thrust the pins into the region of the heart. When he was very busy he could simply draw a target on paper and throw his pen at it imagining that it was a girl. As the years went by he resorted to many other variations. Thus when he lived in the country he would shoulder his rifle and go out into the gadren, and by imagining that he was shooting Indians his bowels were soon stimulated to activity. Sometimes he imagined himself fighting, which gave the same result. On one occasion while throwing his pins at a picture one of them fell through the window into the garden, and as childern were wont to play there, he soon became obsessed with the idea that one of the children might swallow the pin and die. This was the first obsession of this kind and which continued in different forms.

All these patients showed a special interest in their anal activities in childhood and in adult life. Later when the infantile activities of the anal zone remained in a state of repression they belonged to that class of persons who prolong the act of defecation by reading books and newspapers in the water-closet, thus X. referred to the water-closet as his library. With the onset of the neurosis which signified a failure of repression, the originally enhanced anal activities came to the surface in the form of symptoms; *i.e.*, the neurosis represented the negative of the perversion.

The analyses of these as well as of a number of other cases fully corroborate Freud's formula; viz., that the permanent distinguishing traits of a person are either unchanged continuations of the original impulses, sublimations of the same, or reactions formed against them.

REFERENCES

1. Sammlung kleiner Schriften zur Neurosenlehre, 2d Series p. 132.
2. *Cf.* Chap. IV.
3. Freud: Anal Erotic, *l. c.*

CHAPTER XII

FREUD'S THEORY OF WIT

Its Relation to the Dream and Unconscious

When we examine the literature on wit from Aristotle to our present time, we are struck by the fact that despite its universality comparatively little has been written on the subject, and that although many excellent theories have been advanced, notably by Jean Paul, Theodore Vischer, and Fischer, none of these authors has gone deeply enough into the subject.

Without entering into detailed descriptions I shall simply state that the characteristic qualities of wit as given by the most prominent authors are the following: activity, the relation of the content of wit to our thoughts, the character of the playing judgment, the union of dissimilarities, contrasting ideas, sense in nonsense, the succession of confusion and clearness, the sudden emergence of the hidden, and the peculiar kind of brevity.

On close examination it can be readily seen that these qualities though readily demonstrable by many examples of wit represent only isolated fragments, and give us little information about the deeper psychological mechanisms of wit. Indeed no author thoroughly explains the individual determinants of wit. Also the divisions of wit are based by some authors on the technical means, and by others on the usage of wit in speech. The reason for all these diversities and discrepencies is that, with the exception of Freud, no author penetrated deeply enough into the subject. Here, as in some other branches of normal and abnormal psychology Freud pushed on when the others have stopped, and in this book, "Der Witz und sein Beziehung zum Unbewussten,"[1] he solves the riddle of wit as he solved the riddle of the neuroses and psychoses.

Following Freud I have divided this paper into the analytical, synthetical, and theoretical parts.

THE TECHNIQUE OF WIT

DeQuincey once remarked that old persons are apt to fall into "anecdotage." The word *anecdotage*, though in itself incomprehensible, can be readily analysed to show its original full sense; and on analysis we find that it is made up of two words, *anecdote* and *dotage*. That is, instead of saying that old persons are apt to fall into dotage, and that old persons are fond of telling anecdotes, DeQuincey fuses the two words together forming a neologism, *anecdotage*, and thus simultaneously expresses both ideas. The technique, therefore, lies in the fusion of the two words. Such a fusion of words is called *condensation*. Condensation is not a simple composition formed by the joining of the two words; there is a substitutive formation, *i.e.*, instead of *anecdote* and *dotage* we get *anecdotage*.

In a short story that I have recently read, one of the characters, a "sport," speaks of the Christmas season as the *alchoholidays*. By reduction it can be easily seen that we have here a compound word, a combination of *alcohol* and *holidays* which can be graphically represented as follows:

alcoHOL
HOLidays
ALCOHOLIDAYS

Here the condensation expresses the idea that holidays are conducive to alcoholic indulgence. In other words, we have here a fused word, which, though strange in appearance, can be easily understood in its proper context. This witticism may be described as a *condensation with substitution.*

The same mechanism is found in the following: A dramatic critic summarizing three paragraphs to the effect that most plays produced in New York City are violent, emotional and hysterical, remarks, "Thespis has taken up his home in Dramatteawan." The substitution not only expresses the critic's idea that most of the plays at present produced in this city are violent, emotional, and hysterical, that is insane, but it also contains a clever allusion to the nature of the problems presented by most of these plays. Matteawan is a state hospital for criminal insane. Most of the plays are not only insane but also criminal, since they treat of murders, divorces, robberies, scandals, etc.

A jest which not long ago went the rounds in Europe referred to the late King Leopold as Cleopold, on account of his attachment to an actress whose first name was Cleo. This scandalous allusion is here produced by the addition of a single letter.[2]

The examples thus far described come under the group of substitutive formation (Ersatzbildung). Brevity, which Shakespeare calls the soul of wit,[3] is common to them all; but brevity alone is not wit, else every laconism would be wit; it must be a special kind of brevity. Investigation shows that the brevity of the joke is often due to a special process which leaves its definite mark in the wording of the wit. This is the process of substitutive formation. If we apply the process of reduction to the wit, we find that wit depends solely on the verbal expression produced by the process of condensation. As yet, however, we do not understand how the process of condensation produces the most valuable part of wit, namely, the *resultant mirth* (Lustgewinn).

Condensation not only plays a part in wit, but also in dreams. We know that the dream is divided into the manifest and the latent thoughts.[4] The latent thoughts are the actual thoughts underlying the dream, while the manifest thoughts, which are usually absurd and in appearance meaningless, are those which are recalled by the dreamer on awakening. The dream-work is the name given to the psychic processes which are responsible for the transformation of the latent into the manifest thoughts of the dream, and condensation may be named as one of these processes. Words, pictures, ideas, and events are all subject to the process of condensation. It may produce composite pictures resembling one object or person up to a certain ingredient or variation which is drawn from another source. Thus one of my patients saw in her dream a creature resembling a centaur. She soon recognized the head as that of a male acquaintance, but the body, which was that of a horse, presented here a sexual symbolism.[5]

From word condensation we shall now turn to thought condensation, and to illustrate this form the following witticism may be cited. A corporal shouts to his recruits during drill, "Keep it up, boys; courage and perseverance bring everything; the egg of Columbus was not laid in a day."

This jest is formed by the condensation of two separate items—the saying, "Rome was not built in a day," and the anecdote of the egg of Columbus. What the corporal meant to say was, "All that you boys need is practice; it is as simple as it was for Columbus to stand the egg on end; don't be discouraged, Rome was not built in a day." He fused these two ideas, however, and thus produced the substitutive formation, "the egg of Columbus was not laid in a day," which on account of its absurdity and incongruity carries the wit of the jest. Similar mechanisms are found in dreams, but before continuing with our investigation of the analogies between the mechanism of wit and of the dream, we will examine the other processes producing wit.

Hood once remarked that he had to be a lively Hood for a livelihood. As can be readily seen the technique of this witticism is no longer condensation with substitutive formation, as it shows neither an omission nor an abbreviation. The thought is fully expressed as the speaker intended it. "I have to be a lively Hood for a livelihood." What, then, is the technique of this witticism? If we apply our method of reduction we find that the wit remains intact as long as we preserve the name, but that as soon as we replace it by another name, let us say Brown, every trace of wit disappears. This points to the fact that the wit lies in a *twofold application* of the name, first by itself, and then as a suffix. I recall an excellent Italian *jeu d'esprit* of a like nature. At a court ball, in Italy, Napoleon Bonaparte brusquely remarked to a very brilliant lady, "Tutti gli Italiani danzano si male" (all Italians dance so badly), to which she quickly replied, "Non tutti ma buona parte" (Buonaparte). The lady's answer has a double meaning; it may mean, "Not all, but a great many" (buona parte); or the words "buona parte" may be read as one word and then her answer has a totally different significance. It becomes a sharp retort to Napoleon Buonaparte's insulting remark, "Not all Italians dance badly, but Buonaparte does." The wit here lies in the *double application of the name*, first as a whole and then divided in syllables like a charade, thus,

$$\frac{\text{buona parte}}{\text{Buonaparte}}$$

The twofold application of the same words, once as a whole and once divided into syllables, is not the only technique differing from the technique of condensation. There are a great many other ways in which the same word or words may be used in order to serve as a technical means of wit. A witty jest may be produced by using the same words a second time, only slightly changed in their order. The slighter the change the better the technique. The following will illustrate the point:

At a ball in Washington a finished coquette gave Senator

Chauncey M. Depew her fan to hold, and asked him if he could flirt a fan. "No," he replied, "but I can fan a flirt." (New York *Times*, March 13, 1910.) This witty jest was produced by merely changing the order of the words "flirt fan" to "fan flirt." It may also be taken as a good example of repartee.

Oliver Wendell Holmes said, "Put not your trust in money, but put your money in trust." Here, too, the witticism depends mostly on the transposition of the same words.

The manifold application of the same material can be greatly extended if the word or words carrying the wit are used first in one form and then slightly modified. Thus, the old classical saying, "Amantes Amentes" (lovers, lunatics) is an excellent example of this subgroup. The striking similarity between the two words serves to illustrate the close resemblance between love and insanity.

Some words lose their full meaning when used in certain connections, as shown in the following examples. Somebody observed to the younger Charles Mathews that blind persons generally appear contented, and concluded by asking, "How can the blind be happy?" "I suppose," replied Mathews, "they see no reason why they shouldn't." This depends entirely on the word *see* in the last sentence, where it has no longer the full meaning of seeing, but an idiomatic significance equivalent to knowing.

The technique of wit based on *double meaning* forms another subgroup of manifold application. Under this heading we have jests utilizing the double meaning of a name; for example, "No more, Pistol; I would not have you go off here. Discharge yourself of our company, Pistol." (Henry IV, 2.)

Question: "Why have the French rejected Lohengrin?" Answer: "On Elsass's account."[6]

We all know that Cardinal Merry Del Val has been blamed for the awkward Roosevelt-Vatican episode, and the journals the world over have predicted his downfall as the Pope's Secretary of State. The following letter written to the New York *Times*, by Eva S. Rosseau, sums up this popular opinion. "All will be Merry when Del says Val (e) to the Vatican."

The following may be cited as other examples of double meaning. "That Mighty Pen. The superiority of man to nature is continually illustrated. Nature needs an immense quantity of quills to make a goose with, but a man can make a goose of himself with one." (*Christian Register*.)

Here the wit depends entirely on the double meaning of the words *goose* and *quill*, which are first used in their original literal sense and then metaphorically. Double meaning may also be produced by play upon words. Here no violence is done to the word, it is not torn into syllables, nor does the word undergo any modification.

Example: Hostess to her guests: "Make yourselves at home; I always like my guests to be at home." The wit is here produced by the play upon the words *at home*.

A physician, leaving the sick bed of a wife, remarked to the husband, "I don't like her looks." "I haven't liked her looks for some time," was the quick rejoinder of the husband.[7] The physician naturally referred to the condition of the wife, but he expressed his apprehension in such words as to afford the husband the means of utilizing them to assert his conjugal aversion.

There is one thing that strikes us when we examine the various groups described above; they all show a simple and distinct resemblance; they are all special forms of condensation. Thus the manifold application of the same material is nothing but a form of condensation, while the play upon words is merely a condensation without substitutive formation. In other words, all the techniques mentioned above have one characteristic, namely, they all show a tendency toward economy of expression. But, as was said above, we must remember that not every tendency to economize expression is witty. It must possess a special form of economy, upon which the efficiency of the wit depends. But before discussing the question whether the economy mentioned is not counterbalanced by the expenditure of intellectual effort entailed in the formation of such expression, and the question who is the gainer by this economy, we will briefly consider puns.

Puns belong to the lowest form of wit. They can be formed with very little effort. A mere similarity between two words is enough to recall the relationship between the two meanings. Puns may be formed by a similarity of structure, sound, or initial letters. Fischer defines the pun as a bad play on words, because it does not play with the word as a word, but merely as a sound. If we eliminate from the pun the manifold application of the same material, we find that the emphasis lies on the concurrence of the two words serving to make the pun; this is only a subgroup of play upon words. The following will serve as illustrations.

The heading of a poetry column in a daily journal reads, "Verse and Worse."

At a gathering someone spoke disparagingly of a certain drama, and wound up by saying, "It was so poor that the first act had to be rewritten." "And now it is re-rotten," added the punster of the gathering.

In both examples the play is upon the words, not as words, but as sounds.

From the technique of witty words, which we have considered exclusively so far, we will now turn to the technique of witty thoughts, and by way of introduction the following examples will be examined.

Two Jews meet near a bathing establishment. "Have you taken a bath?" asked one. "How is that," answered the other, "is one missing?"[8]

At first sight it would seem that the technique lies in the double meaning of the word *take*. For in the first case the word is used in a colorless idiomatic sense, while in the second it is the verb in its full meaning. This would be a case where the same word is taken now in the empty and now in the full sense, for the wit disappears if instead of using "to take a bath" we should substitute the simple equivalent "to bathe." But on closer examination we find that the reduction has not been applied to the right place. For the jest does not lie in the question, but rather in the answer, that is, in the counter question, "How is that, is one missing?" Provided the sense is not destroyed this answer cannot be robbed of its wit by any dilatation or variation. It is to be noted that in the answer of the second Jew the overlooking of the bath is more significant than the misconception of the word *take*.

In his distress a man borrowed money from a wealthy acquaintance.[9] The same day he was discovered by his creditor in a restaurant eating a dish of salmon with mayonnaise. The creditor reproached him in these words: "You borrow money of me and then order salmon with mayonnaise. Is that what you needed the money for?" "I don't quite understand you," responded the debtor. "When I have no money I cannot eat salmon with mayonnaise, when I have money I am not allowed to eat it. Well, when can I ever eat salmon with mayonnaise?"

Here we no longer discover any double meaning. The repetition of the words "salmon with mayonnaise" is not "a manifold application" of the same material, but an actual, identical repetition required by the content. It may be supposed that the striking thing about the answer is its logical character, but as a matter of fact the answer is illogical. The debtor endeavors to justify himself for spending the borrowed money on luxuries, and asks when he is to be allowed to eat salmon. But this is not a logical question; the creditor does not blame him for eating salmon on the day that he borrows the money, but reminds him that in his condition he has no right to think of such luxuries at all. The poor *bon vivant* disregards this only possible sense of the reproach, and answers about something else, and acts as though he did not understand the reproach. In other words, the answer is deviated from the sense of the reproach.

I could find no examples as good as these two taken from Professor Freud's book to illustrate a new technique of wit, namely, *displacement*. In both the examples mentioned the technique lies in the displacement of the psychic accent. The deviation is especially marked in the bath jest. The first says, "Have you taken a *bath?*" The emphasis lies on the bath element. The second answers as if the question were, "Have you *taken* a bath?" The displacement of the emphasis is made possible only by the wording "taken a bath." The displacement would have been impossible if the question had been, "Have you bathed?" The witless answer would have been, "Bathe? What do you mean? I don't know what that means." The technique of this wit depends on the displacement of the emphasis, from "to bathe" to "to take."

Let us now examine in what relation the technique of displacement stands to the expression of the wit. As shown in the second example (salmon with mayonnaise) the displacement-wit is totally independent of the verbal expression. It does not depend upon words, but on streams of thought. The elimination of the wit cannot be effected by any substitution of words as long as the sense is retained. Reduction is only possible by changing the stream of thought.

Another example of pure displacement is the following:

A rather shabby-looking patient consulted a famous specialist about his malady. After the doctor examined him and gave his opinion he demanded ten dollars, his regular office fee. The patient thought that it was too much, and asked for a reduction. The doctor reduced his fee at first to five and then to three dollars, but the patient persisted that it was still too high a fee for him to pay. The doctor becoming impatient exclaimed, "If you are so poor why did you come to me? You should have gone to a free clinic!" "Nothing is too expensive for my health," responded the patient.

This is certainly in general a proper attitude, but not for this patient. The answer would be proper from the standpoint of a wealthy man who pays his bills without demurring.

The analysis of these examples shows a certain logical elaboration which serves to conceal a displacement of the stream of thought. There are, however, jokes which, instead of logic, display absurdity and nonsense, as the following joke.

A servant girl having been dismissed demands a recommendation from her mistress. The latter refuses to give it, saying, "I cannot recommend you, because you have not kept the house clean. Look at the dust and filth in these corners." "Excuse me, madam," replied the servant, "that is not my fault; that dirt and filth was there when I came a year ago."

The servant's answer is certainly absurd on its face; she attempts to excuse her negligence, but succeeds only in incriminating herself the more. Still, on closer consideration, we find that her answer is not as foolish as it appears; that this nonsense contains sense which turns the nonsense into wit. The servant in giving this answer makes herself appear foolish in order to show her mistress how foolish she herself is. The reduction is as follows: "You blame me for not keeping your house clean; you are no better housekeeper yourself. The dust and filth were in these corners when I came here; and, moreover, what kind of a mistress are you to allow dirt and filth to remain in your house for over a year, and that, too, with a servant in the house! You are very foolish to blame me now."

The technique of this joke consists in advancing something apparently *absurd* and *non-sensical,* which, however, discloses a sense serving to illustrate and represent some further actual absurdity and nonsense.

Besides the examples mentioned in the two groups, namely, of displacement and absurdity, we find other forms of wit showing faulty logic. A good example is the following:

A friend who had stopped in the street to speak to Charles Lamb said to him carelessly as they were parting, "By the way, my dear fellow, you owe me half a crown." "On the contrary," replied Lamb, "it is you who owe me half a crown; for if you will remember, I asked you for five shillings, and you could only lend me two and six." The wit in this anecdote is due to *false logic.* What Lamb says may be true, but it is based on a false premise, as he wrongly assumes that the five shillings were his.

More typical examples of wit based on faulty logic are shown in the three following jokes from the German.

1. A marriage agent is defending the girl he has proposed against the attacks of the prospective fiancé. "I don't like the mother-in-law," the latter remarks; "she is a crabbed, foolish person." "That's true, however, you are not going to marry the mother-in-law, but the daughter." "Yes, but she is no longer young, and she isn't pretty, either." "That's nothing; if she isn't young and pretty you can trust her all the more." "But she hasn't much money." "Why talk of money? Are you marrying money? Don't you want a wife?" "But she's

a hunchback!" "Well, what of that, do you expect her to have no blemishes at all?"[10]

2. On being introduced to his prospective bride, the young man is rather unpleasantly disappointed, and drawing aside the marriage agent, he reproachfully whispers to him, "Why have you brought me here? She is ugly and old, she squints, has bad teeth and bleary eyes! . . . . ." You can talk louder," interposes the marriage agent, "She's deaf, too."[11]

3. The prospective bridegroom makes his first call on the future bride with the marriage agent, and while waiting in the parlor for the appearance of the family, the agent calls the young man's attention to a glass closet containing a handsome silver set. "Just look at these things, you see how wealthy they are." "But isn't it possible," asks the suspicious young man, "that these nice things were borrowed for the occasion in order to give an impression of wealth?" "What an idea," answered the agent, protestingly; "who do you think would lend them anything?"[12]

In joke (1) we have a girl of advanced age, ugly and deformed, who has little money and a repulsive mother, all of which is not very attractive to the young man. The marriage agent knows how to excuse each individual fault, except the inexcusable hunchback, which he must cope with. The girl apparently has many faults which can be overlooked, but one from which you cannot get away, and which is apt to hinder matrimony. The agent acts as if he had removed every individual fault by his excuses, forgetting that each leaves behind some depreciation which accumulates. He insists upon dealing with each factor individually, and refuses to connect them into a whole (sum). The entire joke shows a semblance of logic characteristic of sophism which serves here to conceal the false logic.

The fallacy or sophism in (2) and (3) may be designated as *automatic.* The marriage agent reacts a number of times, one after another, in the same manner, and continues in the same manner on the next occasion when it becomes unsuited and runs contrary to his intentions. Falling into the automatism of habit, he fails to adapt himself to the required situation. Thus the marriage agent in the second story is so fascinated by the failings and infirmities of the bride-to-be that he completes the list from his own knowledge, which it was neither his business nor his intention to do. In the third story he is so carried away by his zeal to convince the young man of the family's wealth, that he comes out with something which upsets all his efforts. In both examples the automatism triumphs over the appropriate variation of thought and expression.

The examples given below take us to another form of the technique of wit.

1. It is called college commencement because the students then commence to forget what they have hitherto learned.

2. If the play is good and the star is rotten,
The author's famous, but the star forgotten.
If the star is good and the play is rotten,
The author gets something, the star gets nothin'!

—*Collier's Irrational Weakly.*

The second example may recall the group of "manifold application of the same material," but in this case as can be readily seen, the double meaning plays no part. The important factors in these examples depend on the formation of new and unexpected identities, and on the production of ideas and definitions related to each other and to a common third. It is a *unification*. Unification is also a basis of the quick repartee in wit, for ready repartee consists in using the defense for aggression, and in "turning the tables," or "in paying with the same coin;" that is, the repartee consists in establishing an unexpected identity between the attack and counter attack. This is well illustrated in the following examples.

A lawyer of small stature came into court to look after his client's interests. His opponent, not knowing him, asked him what he wanted, and on being told who he was, jokingly remarked, "What? Such a little lawyer? Why I could put you into my pocket!" "You could," tranquilly responded the former, "but then you would have more brains in your pocket than in your head."

On returning to Paris after crossing Niagara Falls, Blondin was the hero of the hour. Alexander Dumas, who was one of his many visitors, permitted himself to doubt the feat, upon which Blondin angrily exclaimed, "Well, M. Dumas, if you like, come and walk with me over the Falls." "With pleasure," retorted the celebrated author, "but only on condition that I be allowed to carry you."

The excellent repartee in the last anecdote which meets an impossible demand with just as impossible a condition, contains another technical moment which would be absent if the answer had been, "No, I fear you will not be able to carry me." To illustrate this point I will again quote an example from Freud.

Frederick the Great heard of a clergyman who had the reputation of communicating with spirits. He sent for him and received him with the following question, "Can you call up ghosts?" The answer was, "At your pleasure, your Majesty, but they won't come." Here it is quite obvious that the wit lies in the substitution for the only answer possible, "No," its opposite. To complete this substitution, "but" had to be added to "yes" which gives the equivalent for "No."

Such *representation through the opposite* is another form of technique of wit. A very pure example of this form is the following:

"This woman resembles the Venus de Milo in many points; like her she is extraordinarily old, and has no teeth, and like her she has white spots on the yellow surface of her body" (Heine). Heine thus depicts ugliness by making it agree with the most beautiful.

The following anecdote will serve as another illustration of this group. The great orator, Cicero, once remarked to a man who told him that his wife was thirty years old, "That is undoubtedly true, since I have heard it for the last ten years." What Cicero really meant was, "This cannot be true, as I heard you say the same thing ten years ago." He said just the opposite however, "that is undoubtedly true," and if the next sentence had read, "for I have heard you say this before," it would have merely reinforced the first. Instead it reads, "For I have heard you say this for the last ten years;" that is, he carries the reinforcement too far and thus indicated the opposite of what is expressed in the first part. Cicero thus succeeds in making himself plain by saying the opposite of what he thinks. But this opposite is nothing but a very striking *outdoing*, which forms another group in the technique of wit.

Mrs. A.: "Can you recommend your former servant? Does she understand everything well?" Mrs. B.: "Oh, yes, she understands everything even better."

This is a very simple example of "outdoing" wit. Instead of saying, "No," Mrs. B. says "Yes," and reinforces it with a still stronger affirmative, which, however, thus gives the equivalent for "No."

Besides the technique of expression through the opposite, wit is also produced by expression through the *similar and cognate*, or rather through the homogeneous and coherent. The following story illustrates this group.

An Irishman who was expected to die was visited at the same time by his priest and physician. After they had both performed their functions the dying man turned to the doctor and asked, "Doctor, how much will you charge my wife for your services after I'll be gone?" The doctor was somewhat reluctant to answer, but on being urged he said, "I will ask her for $100." Turning to the priest the Irishman asked the same question, and as he was very insistent the priest answered that he, too, would charge $100 for his services. The Irishman paused for awhile and said, "Doctor, will you please take hold of my right arm, and Father, will you please take hold of my left arm." When they complied with his request he lay back and said, "Now, I can die like the Lord."

The Irishman's remark is quite plain; we deal with a statement which could not be directly expressed. The *indirect expression* in this story was produced in the following manner. The remark, "Now I can die like the Lord," suggested that being between the priest and the doctor recalls the Saviour dying between the two thieves. This involves the suggestion that the speaker, too, is between two thieves. What he really wished to say was, "You are two robbers to charge my wife $100 each." This thought is expressed indirectly by means of association and in a manner designated as *allusion*. This witticism is also an excellent example of the so-called *grim humor* (Galgenhumor).

There are other forms of the technique of wit, but we have described, if only briefly, the most common and most important technical means. These will help us to judge the psychic mechanism and indicate the way for the future solutions of the problem. As mentioned above, the interesting process of condensation with substitution, which we have recognized as the nucleus of the technique of the wit of words, evinces the same mechanism in the formation of dreams. The technique of the wit of thoughts—such as displacement, false logic, absurdity, indirect representation, and expression through the opposite—all these are found also in the technique of dreams. It is displacement that gives the dream its strange appearance and thus prevents us from recognizing in the dream only a continuation of our waking thoughts. The existence of the nonsensical and absurd in the dream is the reason for the belief that there is a deterioration of the psychic activities in the dream, and that the dream shows neither reason nor logic. The popular saying, "Dreams go by contraries," shows well that the idea of expression through the opposite is well known even to the laity. We also find in the dream indirect expressions and the other mechanisms found in wit. All of this shows the close resemblance between the techniques of the dream and of wit, and as will be shown later this resemblance is not at all accidental.

THE TENDENCIES OF WIT

Following the reaction it produces, we divide wit into purposeful, or that which shows definite aims, and harmless, or that which shows no particular aim. It is only the former that is apt to be met with resistances from hearers or persons concerned. There is no relation whatsoever between these classifications and those mentioned above. A harmless joke may be produced by witty words or witty thoughts, and any of the techniques described may serve to produce a purposeful witticism. Following our theoretical explanation of the nature of wit we may say that the harmless wit is for our purposes of greater value than the purposeful, and that the shallow wit is of greater value than the profound. For the harmless and shallow play upon words presents to us the problem of wit in its purest forms, without danger of confusion through the introduction of the tendency factor and consequent false judgment. We often laugh on hearing the most ingenuous and harmless joke where the pleasure experienced cannot have originated from the idea or tendency of the joke; we have then to conclude that the pleasurable feeling is derived from the technique of the wit alone.

The technical means of wit, such as condensation, displacement, indirect expression, etc., have the power of producing in the hearer a feeling of pleasure. We cannot, however, as yet see how they come to possess that power. This gives us a new axiom for the explanation of wit, and brings out more sharply what has been shown above, namely that the character of wit depends on the mode of expression. For it will be recalled that whenever it was possible to reduce the wit by substituting another expression, this not only abrogated the character of the wit, but the laughter-producing effect, that is, the pleasure of the wit. The pleasurable effect of the harmless wit is usually moderate; all that the hearer can expect to obtain from it is a sense of satisfaction and a passing smile; and even this is partially due to the idea. The sudden irresistible outburst of laughter that follows the tendency wit rarely follows the purposeless wit. As the technique is the same in both it may be assumed that by virtue of its tendencies the tendency wit has at its disposal sources of pleasure to which the harmless wit has no access.

Wherever wit is not harmless it serves two tendencies: it is either a hostile joke serving as aggression, satire, or defense, or it is an obscene joke serving as an exhibition.

To examine the way in which wit serves these tendencies we will first discuss the obscene or "smutty" joke. By a "smutty" joke we understand the bringing into prominence of sexual facts or relations through speech. However, a lecture on the anatomy of the sexual organs or on the physiology of reproduction need not necessarily have anything in common with the smutty joke. The smutty joke must fulfil the following condition. It must be directed toward a certain person who excites one sexually, and who becomes cognizant of the speaker's excitement by listening to the smutty joke, and thereby in turn becomes sexually excited. Instead of becoming sexually excited the listener may react with shame and embarrassment, which, however, only shows a reaction against the excitement and thus signifies an admission of the same. The smutty joke was originally directed against the woman, and is comparable to an attempt at seduction. If a man tells or listens to smutty jokes in male society it is because the original situation cannot be realized on account of social inhibitions. The smutty joke is an exhibition directed against a person to whom one is not sexually indifferent. Through the utterance of obscene words the person attacked is incited to picture the parts of the body in question, and is shown that the aggressor pictures the same thing. There is no doubt that the original motive of the smutty joke was the pleasure of seeing the sexual displayed. As shown in the "Three Contributions to the Sexual Theories,"[13] one of the primitive components of our libido is the desire to see the sexual exposed. It is probably only a substitution for the desire to touch the sexual, which is assumed to be the primary pleasure. The libido for looking and touching is found in every person in two forms, active and passive, or masculine and feminine; and in accordance with the preponderance of the sex characteristics it develops preponderately in one or the other direction. At least a certain amount of touching is indispensable in order to attain the normal sexual aim. We all know that touching the skin of the sexual object causes pleasure and excitement. The same holds true of looking, which is analogous to touching. Sexual excitement is frequently awakened by optical impressions, and selection taking account of this fact makes the sexual object a thing of beauty. The covering of the body, which is introduced by civilization, serves to arouse sexual curiosity, and constantly strives to supplement the sexual object by uncovering the hidden parts. This may be turned into the artistic ("sublimation") if the interest be turned from the genitals to the form of the body. The tendency to linger at the intermediary sexual aim by looking is found in most normals. It in a way gives them the capability of directing a certain amount of their libido to a higher artistic aim. But this fondness for looking may become overestimated and fixed, and then becomes a perversion. We then have the so-called *voyeurs* or "peepers." The desire to exhibit is readily observed in children, and where this desire does not experience the sexual repression it develops into a desire for exhibition, a common perversion in grown-up men. In women the passive desire to exhibit is almost regularly covered by the marked reaction of sexual modesty; despite this, however, remnants of the desire may also be seen in women's dress.

In a man a great part of this striving to exhibit remains as a part of the libido, and serves to initiate the sexual act. If the striving asserts itself on first meeting the woman it manifests itself in speech, through which the man makes himself known to woman. By having aroused in her pictures, the woman herself merges into a corresponding excitement, and is thus forced to passive exhibition. The speech of courtship is not regularly the smutty joke, but may pass over into one. If the woman is yielding there is no need for the smutty wit; it is only resorted to when she is resistive and on the defense. As the sexual aggression is inhibited in its progress toward the act, the sexually inciting speech changes into the smutty wit; and the aggressor, lingering at the evocation of the excitement, takes pleasure in the effects his speech produces in the woman. The unyieldingness of the woman is therefore another condition for the determination of the smutty wit. The ideal case for such resistance on the part of the woman usually results from the presence of another man whose presence excludes the immediate yielding of the woman.

The tendency joke usually requires three persons—the first person who makes the wit, the second person who is taken as the object of the hostile or sexual aggression, and the third person in whom the purpose of the wit to produce pleasure is fulfilled. The process may be described as follows: As soon as the libidinous impulse of the first person meets with resistances to his gratification through the woman, he immediately develops a hostile attitude toward this second person and takes the originally intruding third person as his confederate. Through the obscene speech of the first person the woman is exposed before the third person, who as a listener is fascinated by the easy gratification of his own libido. We can now understand what wit performs by its tendency. It makes possible the gratification of a craving (lewd or hostile) despite the hindrance which stands in the way; it eludes the hindrance and draws pleasure from a pleasure source which has become inaccessible through the hindrance. The hindrance in the way is usually nothing but the higher degree of social cultivation which correspondingly increases the inability of the woman to tolerate the bare sexual. The power which renders it difficult or impossible for the woman, and in a lesser degree for the man, to enjoy unveiled obscenities we call "repression." It is the same psychic process which keeps from consciousness whole complexes of emotions and ideas, and has shown itself to be the principal factor in the causation of the psychoneuroses. Civilization and the higher education have helped in the development of this repression, and have produced many changes in our psychic organization. What was once perceived as pleasurable now appears as inacceptable, and is rejected by all the psychic forces. Owing to the repression brought about by civilization many primary pleasures are now disapproved by the censor and lost. But the human psyche finds renunciation difficult, and hence we find that tendency wit gives us the means to make the renunciation retrogressive, and thus regains what has been lost. When we laugh over a delicate obscene witticism we laugh at the same thing which causes laughter in the ill-bred man when he hears a coarse, obscene joke. The pleasure in both cases comes from the same source. The coarse, obscene joke could not, however, incite us to laughter, because it would cause us shame or appear to us disgusting; we can laugh only when wit comes to our aid.[14]

We have now demonstrated what was said at the outset, namely, that the tendency wit has access to other sources of pleasure than the harmless wit, in which all pleasure depends on the technique. We are, however, in no position to distinguish in the tendency wit what part of the pleasure originates from the technique and what part from the tendency. Strictly speaking, we do not know over what we are laughing.

When we examine the rôle of wit in the service of the hostile tendency we at once meet with similar conditions. Since our individual childhood and the childhood of human civilization our hostile impulses toward our fellow beings, like our sexual strivings, have been subjected to restrictions and repressions. Even to-day we are not yet ready to love our enemies and to extend to them our left cheek after we are smitten on the right. Nevertheless, we have made some progress in controlling our hostile feelings. Higher civilization and culture trains us to suppress the hostile disposition; we are taught that it is undignified to use insulting language, and even the means of combat have been markedly restricted. Society as the third person in the combat, for the protection of its own interest, prevents us from expressing our hostile feelings in action; and hence, as in the sexual aggression, there has developed a new technique of invective, the aim of which is to enlist the third person against our enemy. By belittling and humbling our enemy, by scorning and ridiculing him, we indirectly obtain the pleasure of his defeat through the laughter of the third person, the passive spectator.

The wit of hostile aggression gives us the means to make our enemy ridiculous, which, on account of the existing hindrances, could not be effected in any other way; in other words, wit affords us the means of surmounting the restrictions and of opening the otherwise inaccessible pleasure sources. Because of the gain in pleasure it fascinates the hearer to take our part, even if he is not convinced—just as we are wont to overestimate the substance of witty remarks when we are fascinated by their technique. By way of illustration the following example may be cited: Wendell Phillips, according to the recent biography by Dr. Lorenzo Sears, was, on one occasion, lecturing in Ohio, and while on a railroad journey going to keep one of his appointments, he met in the car a number of clergymen returning from some sort of convention. One of the ministers felt called upon to approach Mr. Phillips, and asked him, "Are you Mr. Phillips?" "I am, sir." "Are you trying to free the niggers?" "Yes, sir; I am an abolitionist." "Well, why do you preach your doctrines up here? Why don't you go over into Kentucky?" "Excuse me, are you a preacher?" "I am, sir." "Are you trying to save souls from hell?" "Yes, sir, that's my business." "Well, why don't you go there?" The assailant hurried into the smoker amid a roar of unsanctified laughter. This anecdote nicely illustrates the tendency wit in the service of hostile aggression. The minister's behavior was offensive and irritating, yet Wendell Phillips as a man of culture could not defend himself in the same manner as a common ill-bred person would have done, and as his inner feelings must have prompted him to do. The only alternative under the circumstances would have been to take the affront in silence, had not wit showed him the way, and enabled him by the technical means of unification to turn the tables on his assailant. He not only belittled him and turned him into ridicule, but by his clever retort, "Well, why don't you go there?" fascinated the other clergymen, and thus brought them to his side. The anecdote of the two lawyers mentioned above shows the same mechanism.

We have now shown that the pleasure found in wit is produced on the one hand by the technique, and on the other hand by the tendency. We will next endeavor to discover the common source uniting both.

THE PLEASURE MECHANISM AND PSYCHOGENESIS OF WIT

In endeavoring to discover how the pleasure results from the technique and the tendency of wit, and the mechanism of this resulting pleasure, we find that the explanation sought for can be more readily discovered in the tendency than in the harmless wit. That the pleasure in the tendency wit results from the gratification of a tendency, which gratification would not otherwise take place, is quite obvious. But the manner in which wit produces this gratification depends on special determinations. There are two different cases to be considered. The simpler of the two is the case in which an outer hindrance stands in the way of the gratification of the tendency. This may be illustrated by the following example: "How many members are there in your council of ten?" Louis XIV once sarcastically asked the embassador of the republic of Venice. "Forty, your Majesty," retorted the polite Italian. The wit in this case serves to return one affront for another. The ambassador could not answer as he would have liked, because Louis XIV could not be insulted, so he skilfully made use of the unification wit, and thus paid him in his own coin.

The second class comprises cases in which internal hindrances stand in the way of the direct realization of the tendency. As examples we may cite the answer of the lawyer to his opponent, and Wendell Phillips's answer to the clergyman. Wendell Phillips was prevented from using invectives by a highly developed esthetic sense, but wit helped to overcome the inner resistances and to remove the inhibitions. The gratification of the tendency is made possible, and in this way the suppression and the "psychic damming" connected with it is evaded. The mechanism of the development of pleasure is the same in both cases. The only difference between the cases of outer and inner hindrances consists in the fact that in the one an already existing inhibition is removed, while in the other the formation of a new inhibition is evaded. We may add that the formation as well as the retention of a psychic inhibition necessitates a "psychic expenditure." If pleasure is obtained in the employment of both kinds of the tendency wit, it may be readily assumed *that such resultant pleasure corresponds to the economy of psychic expenditure.*

Again we are confronted with the principle of *economy* first noticed in the technique of the wit of words; but whereas the economy was there confined to the use of few or possibly the same words, it seems here to comprise the economy of psychic expenditure in general. The secret of the pleasure secured through tendency wit seems to be in the economy of the expenditure of inhibition or suppression. We shall now turn to the mechanism of the pleasure of the harmless wit.

In examining appropriate examples of harmless wit we

concluded that the source of pleasure lies solely in the technique of the wit. Let us now see whether this pleasure can be traced to an economy of psychic expenditure.

The technique of one group of this wit, the play upon words, consisted in directing the psychic focus on the sound instead of on the sense of the word, which greatly facilitated the psychic labor. It is known that in abnormal mental states where the possibility of concentrating psychic expenditure on one place is reduced, the word sounds are more prominent than their significance, and that such patients react with "outer" instead of "inner" associations.[15] Children who still treat the word as an object, show a tendency to seek the same sense under the same or similar wording. This provides no small amount of amusement for grown-ups. If wit gives us pleasure by employing the same or similar words in order to reach from one idea to another, we can justly say that this pleasure is due to the economy of psychic expenditure.

A second group of technical means of wit—unification, accordance, allusions and citations—all these evince one common character; namely, one always discovers something familiar when one expects instead something new. To discover the familiar is pleasurable. It is not difficult to recognize such pleasure as one of economy and to refer it to the economy of psychic expenditure. That recognition of the familiar causes pleasure is universally admitted. We know also that the source of pleasure in rhyme, alliteration, refrain, and other forms of repetition of similar sounding words in poetry, is due merely to the discovery of the familiar.

It may be thought at first sight that the third group in

the technique, viz., wit of thought, which includes displacement, false logic, absurdity, representation through the opposite, etc., bears no relation to the technique of discovering the familiar, but it will not be difficult to demonstrate that this group, too, shows an economy or facilitation of psychic expenditure. It is quite obvious that it is easier to turn away from a definite trend of thought than to stick to it; it is easier to mix up different things than to distinguish them; and it is particularly easier to pass over illogical conclusions. Moreover, in connecting words or thoughts it is especially easy to overlook the fact that such connections should result in sense. These mechanisms are well known and are those especially used in the techniques of the wit mentioned above. It will sound strange, however, to assert that such processes in the work of wit may produce pleasure.

Though "pleasure and nonsense" is almost absent in our serious existence it can still be demonstrated in two cases. It is visible in the learning child, and in the adult under toxic influences. When the child learns to have command over its mother tongue it takes pleasure in playing with words. It disregards the meaning of the words and connects them in order to obtain pleasure through rhythm and rhyme. An excellent example of this is the familiar "Mother Goose." As the child becomes older it is forced to abandon this pleasure and to employ the words in their senseful meaning. But even later in life there is a tendency to overstep the restrictions in the use of words, and adults often change words by adding suffixes and prefixes and reduplications. This is especially seen in the neologisms of the insane.[16]

The child makes use of play in order to withdraw from the pressure of critical reason which is imposed upon it in the course of development. The restrictions appear still greater when in the education of right thinking it becomes necessary to separate reality from fiction. As a persistent resistance against these restrictions we may mention the formation of fancies. The force of reason becomes so strong in later childhood and puberty that the child then rarely dares to utter nonsense. But men are untiring pleasure seekers, and find it extremely difficult to renounce pleasure once experienced. The tendency to skylarking in students is nothing but a demonstration against the tyranny of forced study and reality, which they tolerate only impatiently. No one can fail to recognize in our college cries and songs the nonsensical and infantile play with words. These feelings are especially enhanced by alcoholic indulgence under which influence the grown up again becomes a child. He derives pleasure from a free disposal of his mental stream which is now unencumbered by the restraint of logic.

In reviewing the three groups of the technique of wit it has been shown that the technique of the absurd corresponds to a source of pleasure; and that this pleasure is produced by the economy of psychic expenditure, and by the relief from the restraint of reason. When we traced the psychogenesis of wit we found that the first step in wit is play. The child plays when it learns to use words and connect thoughts, and this playing is probably the result of an impulse which urges the child to exercise its capacities (Groos). Through the repetition of similarities, the rediscovering of the familiar, and sound associations, it obtains pleasure which may be explained as an unexpected economy of psychic expenditure. But this playing is later brought to an end by reason which rejects it as senseless or absurd. It is only accidentally that the grown up finds pleasure in the rediscovering of the familiar. This only occurs when he is in a playful mood, which, as in the child, removes the critical inhibitions. But as men do not like to wait for these propitious occasions, and also hate to forego this pleasure, they seek means to make themselves independent of these pleasant states. This effort to evade reason and find a substitute for the pleasant mood produces the second element of wit, the jest.

The object of the jest is to bring about the resultant pleasure of playing, and at the same time appease the protesting reason which strives to suppress the pleasant feeling. The only way to accomplish this is to give sense and meaning to the senseless and absurd combination of words or thoughts. The whole process of wit production is therefore directed toward the discovery of word and thought constellations which fulfil these conditions. The jest makes use of almost all the technical means of wit. The most conspicuous factor of the jest is the gratification it affords by making possible that which reason forbids. Its object is to remove inner inhibitions and thereby to render productive those pleasure sources which have become inaccessible.

If we follow the development of the jest until it reaches its height in the tendency wit we find that the jest's effort is to produce pleasure and that it is content when its utterance does not appear perfectly senseless or insipid. If this utterance is substantial and valuable it changes into wit. When we hear a good witticism we experience a general feeling of satisfaction without being able to tell at once what part of the pleasure comes from the witty form, and what part from the excellent thought. We really do not know what gives us the pleasure and at what we are laughing. This uncertainty of our judgment may have given the motive for the formation of the wit in the literal sense. The thought seeks the disguise of wit, because through the wit it recommends itself to our attention and can appear to us more important and valuable than it is, but above all because this disguise fascinates and confuses our reason. We are apt to attribute to the thought the pleasure derived from the witty form, and we are not inclined to consider improper what gives us pleasure, and in this way to close up a source of pleasure. For if wit makes us laugh it is because it establishes in us a disposition unfavorable to reason and conducive to play. To accomplish this the wit had to exert all its effort. Although such wit is harmless, and not purposeful, we can assume that strictly speaking the jest alone shows no tendency, that is, it serves to produce pleasure only. Wit, on the other hand, is never purposeless, as the great tendencies and impulses of our psychic life use it for their purposes. We have shown above the part played by wit in satisfying the hostile and obscene impulses; the hostile wit changes the original indifferent hearers into haters and scorners, and thus confronts the enemy with an army of opponents where there was formerly but one. The obscene wit makes a confederate of the third person, who originally disturbed the sexual situation, by giving him pleasure through the utterance which causes the woman to be ashamed in his presence. In the first case wit overthrows the critical judgment which would have otherwise examined the dispute in question, while in the second case it overcomes the inhibitions of shame and decorum by the pleasure premium which it offers.

What impressed us most on first reviewing the processes of the tendency wit was the effect it produced on the hearer. It is more important, however, to understand the effect produced by wit on the psychic life of the person who makes it, or, to be more precise, in the person who conceives it.

In regard to its distribution we may study the psychic processes of wit in reference to two persons, the wit producer and the hearer. We can at present assume that the psychic process aroused by wit in the hearer is usually an imitation of the psychic processes of the wit producer. The outer inhibitions which are overcome in the hearer correspond to the inner inhibitions of the wit producer. Of the different forms of the inner inhibitions one especially merits consideration. We designate that form by the name of "repression," and it is characterized by the fact that it excludes from consciousness certain former emotions and their products. Tendency wit is capable of liberating pleasure from sources which have undergone repression. If the overcoming of outer hindrances can be traced to inner inhibitions and repressions we may say that the tendency wit proves more clearly than any other developmental stage of wit that the main character of wit-making is to set free pleasure by removing inhibitions. The tendency wit reinforces the tendencies which it serves by bringing to them assistance from repressed emotions or it serves directly the repressed tendencies. Although we may readily assert that these are the functions of the tendency wit, we must also admit that we cannot understand in what manner these actions can succeed. This is a rather complicated process which we will attempt to demonstrate synthetically.

According to G. Th. Fechner, a meeting of pleasurable conditions will produce a resultant pleasure greater than the sum of the pleasure values of the separate conditions. The result is greater than the sum total of the single effects. The theme of wit does not give us the opportunity to test the correctness of this principle. But from wit we have learned something else which at least comes near this principle. We have shown above that in a cooperatoin of many pleasure-producing factors we are in no position to assign to each one the resultant part which really belongs to it. But the situation assumed in the principle of assistance can be varied, and for these new conditions we can formulate the following questions and answers: What happens if in one constellation there is a meeting of pleasurable and painful conditions? Upon what depends the result and the previous indications of the same? The tendency wit particularly shows these possibilities. There is one tendency which strives to liberate pleasure from a certain source, while there is another which works against this pleasurable development, that is, which inhibits or suppresses it. The suppressing stream, as the result shows, must be somewhat stronger than the one suppressed, and is therefore not abolished. But now there appears a second tendency which would strive to set free pleasure by the same process though from a different source; it thus acts like the suppressed one. What can be the result? This will be better illustrated by an example. There is a tendency to insult a certain person, but against this there is a feeling of decorum and esthetic culture. If by virtue of some emotional state the insult should happen to break through it would subsequently be painfully perceived. The insult is therefore omitted. There is a possibility, however, of making good wit from the words or thoughts which would have served in the insult, that is, pleasure can be set free from other sources without being hindered by the same suppression. But the second development of pleasure would have to be omitted if the insulting were not admitted, and as the latter is admitted it is connected with the new liberation of pleasure. Experience with tendency wit shows that under such circumstances the suppressed tendency can become so strengthened by the help of wit pleasure as to overcome the otherwise stronger inhibition. But the satisfaction thus obtained is not produced by the wit alone; it is incomparably greater, in fact it is by so much greater than the pleasure of the wit that we must assume that the former suppressed tendency has succeeded in breaking through, perhaps without an outlet. Under these conditions the tendency wit causes the most prolific laughter. Hence we see that the case of the tendency wit is a special case of the principle of help. A possibility of the development of pleasure enters into a situation in which another possibility of pleasure is hindered so that this alone would not result in pleasure. The result is a development of pleasure which is greater by far than the entering possibility. The latter acted, as it were, as an alluring premium, and with the aid of a small sum of pleasure a very large sum is obtained. The pleasure serving to liberate the large sum of pleasure is designated as *fore-pleasure* (Vorlust), and the principle is designated as the principle of fore-pleasure.

The effect of the tendency wit can be formulated as follows: It enters into the service of tendencies in order to produce new pleasure by removing suppressions and repressions. This it does by means of the wit pleasure as fore-pleasure. When we review its development we find that it begins as play in order to produce pleasure from the free use of words and thoughts. When the growing reason forbids this senseless play with words and thoughts it turns to the jest or joke in order to hold on to these pleasure sources, and in order to be able to gain new pleasure from the liberation of the absurd. As harmless wit it assists thoughts and enforces them against the impugnment of critical judgment. In this it makes use of the principle of confounding the pleasure sources. It finally enters into the great struggling suppressed tendencies in order to remove inner inhibitions in accordance with the principle of fore-pleasure. It combats in turn the reason—the critical judgment—and the repression. It firmly adheres to the original word pleasure sources, and opens new pleasure sources by removing inhibitions. The pleasure which it produces, be it play-pleasure or removal-pleasure, can at all time be traced to the economy of psychic expenditure.

THE MOTIVES OF WIT AND WIT AS A SOCIAL PROCESS

Although the desire to gain pleasure is clearly a sufficient motive of wit, there are other motives which may participate in its production. Though wit-making is an excellent means of obtaining pleasure from the psychic processes, we know that not all persons are equally able to make use of it. Wit making is not at the disposal of everybody; indeed few persons seem to possess this gift. It is entirely independent of intelligence, phantasy, memory, etc. A special talent or psychic determination permitting or favoring wit making must be presupposed in all wits. It is not often possible to investigate this theme; only now and then can we enter into the subjective determinations in the mind of the wit maker. The physician indeed occasionally has opportuntiy to study persons who, if not renowned wits, are recognized in their circle as witty; and he is often surprised to find such persons showing dissociated personalities and a predisposition to nervous affections. Owing, however, to insufficient investigations this cannot be put down as a general rule. A clearer case is afforded by jokes of Jewish subject-matter, and made exclusively by Jews. The determination for the self-participation seems to be plain. It is due to the fact that the person finds it difficult to directly express his criticism and aggression and is thus compelled to resort to byways. Jewish jokes not produced by Jews never rise above the level of the comical strain or the brutal mockery. The motive for the production of harmless wit is usually the ambitious impulse "to show off," or to give a favorable impression. It is an impulse comparable to the sexual exhibition. The existence of numerous inhibited impulses, the suppression of which retains a certain degree of liability, produces a state favorable for the production of the tendency wit. Certain components of the sexual constitution may appear as motives for wit formation. Persons inclined to obscene joking usually conceal a desire to exhibit. Persons having a powerful sadistic component in their sexuality, which is more or less inhibited, are most successful with the tendency wit of aggression. It is universally known that no person is satisfied with making wit for himself. Wit making is inseparably connected with the desire to impart it. To impart the comical to another person is pleasurable, but one can enjoy it alone, while wit must be imparted. Apparently the psychic process of wit formation does not end with the conception of the wit. There is something left which strives to complete the mysterious process of wit formation by imparting it. The wit producer is in need of another person to whom the wit may be imparted. Wit is thus a social process. Due to the wit making, the person who makes the wit does not laugh at his own production, but he causes inhibitions to become superfluous in the hearer and thus cause a discharge of the repression of the hearer through laughter. The hearer may be said to laugh with the amount of psychic energy which is set free by the suspension of inhibitions; that is, we laugh away, as it were, this amount of psychic energy. When we laugh at a joke we really do not know what we are laughing at; this can be ascertained by analysis. Laughing is the result of an automatic process and is possible only in the absence of conscious attention. It is the property of wit to exert its full effect on the hearer only when it is new and surprising to him. This property, which causes wit to be shortlived, and forever urges the production of new wit, is apparently due to the fact that it is in the nature of the surprising and the unexpected not to succeed a second time. When we repeat wit the awakened memory leads the attention to the first hearing. This also explains the desire to impart wit to others who have not heard it before, for the impression made by wit on the new hearer replenishes in the wit maker that part of the pleasure which has been lost by the lack of novelty. An analogous motive probably urges the wit producer to impart his wit to others.

THE RELATION OF WIT TO DREAMS AND TO THE UNCONSCIOUS

It is to be regretted that we cannot here enter fully into the deep psychological mechanisms of dreams, which are so essential to illustrate the similar mechanisms of wit. I will have to refer the reader to the last chapter of Freud's Interpretation of Dreams. We may however attempt to show some of the profounder relations between the dream and wit.

Besides the resemblances in the techniques of wit and dreams—condensation, displacement, and so on—we also find that the formation of wit is similar to the formation of dreams; that is, *a fore-conscious thought is left for a moment to the unconscious elaboration and its result is forthwith grasped by the conscious perception.* Like the dream, wit is an involuntary mental occurrence. One cannot tell a moment before what joke he is going to crack. One usually experiences something indefinable which Prof. Freud compares to an absence or sudden suspension of intellectual tension, and the wit then appears suddenly. Brevity, too, is common to both wit and dreams. In both this is the result of the process of condensation. The thought which merges into the unconscious for the purpose of forming wit seeks there the infantile play with words, for the infantile is the source of the unconscious. The thought is put back for a moment into the infantile stage in order to regain possession of the childish pleasure sources. As has already been demonstrated in the psychology of the neuroses the peculiar elaboration of wit is only an infantile type of thinking. The dream, also, wherein the child with all its impulses continues to live, has its origin in the infantile life.

Besides the many resemblances between dreams and wit we can also discover some differences. The most important difference lies in their social behavior. The dream is a perfect asocial psychic product; having originated in a person as a compromise between struggling psychic streams, it remains incomprehensible to the person himself, and has no interest or information for anybody else. Wit, on the other hand, is the most social of all the psychic functions aiming to gain pleasure; it often requires three persons, and the psychic process which it incites always requires the participation of at least one other person. The dream is a hidden wish, while wit is a developed play. Despite all its apparent unreality the dream retains its relation to the important practical interests of life; it seeks to fulfill the needs through a regressive detour of hallucinations, and it owes its existence to the strong need for sleep during the night. Wit, on the other hand, seeks to draw a small amount of pleasure from the free activities of our psychic apparatus, and to seize this pleasure as an incidental gain. It thus secondarily reaches to important functions relative to the outer world. The dream serves preponderately to guard from pain, while wit serves to acquire pleasure, but all our psychic activities meet in these two aims.

WIT AND THE COMIC

Comic differs from wit in its social behavior. The comic is content with only two persons, one who finds the comical and one in whom it is found. A third person to whom the comical may be imparted reinforces the comic process, but adds nothing new to it. In wit the third person is indispensable for the protection of the pleasure-bearing process, while the second person may be omitted, especially when we do not deal with tendency and aggressive wit. Wit is made, while the comical is found. The comic is usually found first in persons, and later by transference it may be seen also in objects, situations, etc. We also know that wit occasionally reopens inaccessible sources of the comic, and that the comic often serves to wit as a façade to replace the fore-pleasure.

That form of comic which is nearest to wit is the naive or ingenuous. The naive, like the comic, is usually found and not made. It must result without our intervention from the speech and actions of other persons, and it can only be produced by persons who have no inhibitions to overcome. What conditions the functions of the naive is the fact that we are aware that the person does not possess this inhibition; otherwise we should not call it naive, but impudent, and instead of laughing we should be indignant. The effect of the naive which is irresistible, seems easy to understand. The inhibition which is usually formed in us suddenly becomes inapplicable when we hear the naive, and is discharged through laughing. As the removal of the inhibition is direct, and not the result of an incited operation, there is no need for a suspension of attention. We behave like the hearer in wit, to whom the economy of inhibition is given without any effort on his part. The naive is mostly found in children in whom no inhibitions are developed and in uneducated adults, whom we consider as children in reference to their intellectual development. The following examples will serve as illustrations.

Little Boy: "I want the doctor to come to our house." Servant: "Where do you come from?" Little Boy: "Don't you know me? Why, we do business with you; we had a baby from here last week."

Said a farmer: "I understand that they make instruments with which the stars and planets can be examined. That I know is possible; but how the learned men discovered the names of the stars and planets—that I cannot understand."

The examples of naiveté do not apparently differ from wit in either structure or technique. It is merely a question whether the speaker intends to be witty, or whether, owing to his uncorrected ignorance, he is serious or means precisely what he says. In the latter case we deal with the naive. The naive agrees with wit in both structure and content, but the psychic process of the first person or producer, which is so interesting in wit, is here entirely absent. The ingenuous person imagines that he is using his thoughts and expressions in a simple and normal manner; he has no other purpose in view, and receives no pleasure from his naive productions. Thus the little boy believed that children are obtained from the doctor, and the farmer actually thought that every star and planet comes into existence with a definite name, which men of science have a way of discovering. All the characters of the naive lie in the conception of the hearer, who corresponds to the third person of the wit. The producing person creates the naive without any effort. The complicated technique which in wit serves to paralyze the inhibition produced by the critical reason does not exist here, because the person does not yet possess this inhibition, and he can therefore readily produce the senseless and the obscene without any compromise.

We have said above that the effective determination of wit consists in the fact that both persons should be subjected to about the same inhibition of inner resistances; we may say now that the determination of the naive consists in the fact that one person should have inhibitions which the other lacks. It is the person provided with inhibitions who understands the naive, and it is he alone who gains the pleasure produced by the naive. This, as we know, is due to the removal of inhibitions. But in order to recognize the naive we have to be cognizant of the fact that there are no inner inhibitions in the producing persons. It is only when this is assured that we laugh, instead of being indignant. We take into consideration the psychic state of the producing person; we imagine ourselves in the same, and endeavor to understand it by comparing it to our own psychic state. This putting ourselves into the psychic state of the producing person and comparing it with our own results in an economy of expenditure which we discharge through laughing. This strange mechanism is perhaps the essential part of the psychic process of the comic. Looking at it from this viewpoint the naive is a form of the comic. The pleasure produced by the naive is "comical" pleasure. It originates through an economy of expenditure by comparing the utterances of some one else with our own. The comical, therefore, results in an unintentional discovery in the social relations of men. It is found in persons, that is, in their movements, shapes, actions, etc., and sometimes also in animals and inanimate objects.

The comical can be removed from the person in whom it is found if the condition under which a person becomes comical can be recognized. This shows that there is a comical situation into which any person can place himself or others to appear comical. The means which can effect this are: transference into comic situations, imitation, disguise, unmasking, caricature, parody, travesty, etc. As can be seen, the sphere of origin for the comic is considerably broader than that of the naive. In order to trace the determination of the comic we will examine the comic movement.

We laugh at the actions of clowns because they appear to us immoderate and inappropriate, that is, we really laugh over the excessive expenditure. The child's emotions do not appear to us comical even if it jumps and fidgets, but it is comical to see a little boy follow with his tongue the movements of his pen when he is trying to master the art of writing. We see in this additional motion a superfluous expenditure of energy which we should save under similar conditions. In the same way we find it comical to see a marked exaggeration of expressive motions in adults. Thus we laugh at grimaces which exaggerate the normal expressions of emotions, even if they are involuntary, as in chorea and tics. We laugh because we compare the motions observed in others with those which we ourselves should produce if we were in their place. That person appears to us comical who puts forth too much expenditure in his physical functions and too little in his psychic. Our laughing in both cases expresses a pleasant feeling of superiority which we attribute to ourselves when we compare ourselves with him. This is one of the most important factors in the genesis of the comic.

The difference between the comic and wit is found in the chief psychological character of the comic. The pleasure source of wit we have found in the unconscious, but there is no reason for the same localization of the comic. On the contrary, all the analyses point to the fact that the source of the comical pleasure is the comparison of two expenditures which we must attribute to the fore-conscious. The main difference between wit and comic is found in the psychic localization; wit is, so to say, the contribution of the comic from the sphere of the unconscious.

Without entering into the details of other forms of the

comic we will briefly discuss humor. Humor is the means of obtaining pleasure despite existing painful effects. If we are in a situation which causes us to liberate painful affects, and motives then urge us to suppress the same in statu nascendi, we have the conditions for humor. Thus persons afflicted with misfortune, pain, etc., can gain humoristic pleasure while the onlookers laugh over the comical pleasure. The pleasure of humor results at the cost of this discontinued liberation of affect; it originates through an economy of emotional expenditure. Humor does not require the participation of another person; one can enjoy the pleasure of humor without feeling the necessity of imparting it to another. To understand the psychological mechanisms of humoristic pleasure it is best to examine the so-called "grim humor" (Galgenhumor), where we regularly find that humor is produced at the cost of a great expenditure of psychic work. Economy of sympathy is one of the most frequent causes of humoristic pleasure. Mark Twain's humor usually shows this mechanism.

Humor stands nearer to the comic than wit. Like the comic it is located in the fore-conscious, whereas wit is formed as a compromise between the unconscious and fore-conscious.

We have shown that the pleasure of wit originates from an economy of expenditure in inhibition, of the comic from an economy of expenditure in thought, and of humor from an economy of expenditure in feeling. All three activities of our psychic apparatus derive pleasure from economy. They all strive to bring back from the psychic activity a pleasure which has been lost in the development of this activity; for the euphoria which we are thus striving to obtain is nothing but the state of a bygone time in which we were wont to defray our psychic work with slight expenditure. It is the state of our childhood in which we did not know the comic, were incapable of wit, and did not need humor to make us happy.

References

1. An English translation in preparation.
2. Freud: *L. c.*, p. 12.
3. Hamlet, Act II, Scene II, 1.90.
4. The Interpretation of Dreams. George Allen Co., London, and The Macmillan Co., New York. *Cf.* also Chap. II.
5. *Cf.* Chap. II.
6. Freud: *L. c.*, p. 25.
7. Freud: *L. c.*, p. 26.
8. Freud: *L. c.*, p. 36.
9. Freud: *L. c.*, p. 37.
10. Freud: *L. c.*, p. 47.
11. Freud: *L. c.*, p. 50.
12. Freud: *L. c.*, p. 50.
13. Translated by A. A. Brill, Journal of Nervous and Mental Diseases. Monograph series, No. 7.
14. *Cf.* Chap. II, p. 44. The obscene joke formed by the sound associations bald-balled fulfils all the conditions of the purposive smutty joke.
15. *Cf.* Chap. V.
16. *Cf.* Chap. V.

INDEX

Medicine & Society In America

An Arno Press/New York Times Collection

Alcott, William A. **The Physiology of Marriage.** 1866. New Introduction by Charles E. Rosenberg.

Beard, George M. **American Nervousness:** Its Causes and Consequences. 1881. New Introduction by Charles E. Rosenberg.

Beard, George M. **Sexual Neurasthenia.** 5th edition. 1898.

Beecher, Catharine E. **Letters to the People on Health and Happiness.** 1855.

Blackwell, Elizabeth. **Essays in Medical Sociology.** 1902. Two volumes in one.

Blanton, Wyndham B. **Medicine in Virginia in the Seventeenth Century.** 1930.

Bowditch, Henry I. **Public Hygiene in America.** 1877.

Bowditch, N[athaniel] I. **A History of the Massachusetts General Hospital:** To August 5, 1851. 2nd edition. 1872.

Brill, A. A. **Psychanalysis:** Its Theories and Practical Application. 1913.

Cabot, Richard C. **Social Work:** Essays on the Meeting-Ground of Doctor and Social Worker. 1919.

Cathell, D. W. **The Physician Himself and What He Should Add to His Scientific Acquirements.** 2nd edition. 1882. New Introduction by Charles E. Rosenberg.

The Cholera Bulletin. Conducted by an Association of Physicians. Vol. I: Nos. 1–24. 1832. All published. New Introduction by Charles E. Rosenberg.

Clarke, Edward H. **Sex in Education;** or, A Fair Chance for the Girls. 1873.

Committee on the Costs of Medical Care. **Medical Care for the American People:** The Final Report of The Committee on the Costs of Medical Care, No. 28. [1932].

Currie, William. **An Historical Account of the Climates and Diseases of the United States of America.** 1792.

Davenport, Charles Benedict. **Heredity in Relation to Eugenics.** 1911. New Introduction by Charles E. Rosenberg.

Davis, Michael M. **Paying Your Sickness Bills.** 1931.

Disease and Society in Provincial Massachusetts: Collected Accounts, 1736–1939. 1972.

Earle, Pliny. **The Curability of Insanity:** A Series of Studies. 1887.

Falk, I. S., C. Rufus Rorem, and Martha D. Ring. **The Costs of Medical Care:** A Summary of Investigations on The Economic Aspects of the Prevention and Care of Illness, No. 27. 1933.

Faust, Bernhard C. **Catechism of Health:** For the Use of Schools, and for Domestic Instruction. 1794.

Flexner, Abraham. **Medical Education in the United States and Canada:** A Report to The Carnegie Foundation for the Advancement of Teaching, Bulletin Number Four. 1910.

Gross, Samuel D. **Autobiography of Samuel D. Gross, M.D.,** with Sketches of His Contemporaries. Two volumes. 1887.

Hooker, Worthington. **Physician and Patient;** or, A Practical View of the Mutual Duties, Relations and Interests of the Medical Profession and the Community. 1849.

Howe, S. G. **On the Causes of Idiocy.** 1858.

Jackson, James. **A Memoir of James Jackson, Jr., M.D.** 1835.

Jennings, Samuel K. **The Married Lady's Companion, or Poor Man's Friend.** 2nd edition. 1808.

The Maternal Physician; a Treatise on the Nurture and Management of Infants, from the Birth until Two Years Old. 2nd edition. 1818. New Introduction by Charles E. Rosenberg.

Mathews, Joseph McDowell. **How to Succeed in the Practice of Medicine.** 1905.

McCready, Benjamin W. **On the Influences of Trades, Professions, and Occupations in the United States, in the Production of Disease.** 1943.

Mitchell, S. Weir. **Doctor and Patient.** 1888.

Nichols, T[homas] L. **Esoteric Anthropology:** The Mysteries of Man. [1853].

Origins of Public Health in America: Selected Essays, 1820–1855. 1972.

Osler, Sir William. **The Evolution of Modern Medicine.** 1922.

The Physician and Child-Rearing: Two Guides, 1809–1894. 1972.

Rosen, George. **The Specialization of Medicine:** with Particular Reference to Ophthalmology. 1944.

Royce, Samuel. **Deterioration and Race Education.** 1878.

Rush, Benjamin. **Medical Inquiries and Observations.** Four volumes in two. 4th edition. 1815.

Shattuck, Lemuel, Nathaniel P. Banks, Jr., and Jehiel Abbott. **Report of a General Plan for the Promotion of Public and Personal Health.** Massachusetts Sanitary Commission. 1850.

Smith, Stephen. **Doctor in Medicine** and Other Papers on Professional Subjects. 1872.

Still, Andrew T. **Autobiography of Andrew T. Still,** with a History of the Discovery and Development of the Science of Osteopathy. 1897.

Storer, Horatio Robinson. **The Causation, Course, and Treatment of Reflex Insanity in Women.** 1871.

Sydenstricker, Edgar. **Health and Environment.** 1933.

Thomson, Samuel. **A Narrative, of the Life and Medical Discoveries of Samuel Thomson.** 1822.

Ticknor, Caleb. **The Philosophy of Living;** or, The Way to Enjoy Life and Its Comforts. 1836.

U.S. Sanitary Commission. **The Sanitary Commission of the United States Army:** A Succinct Narrative of Its Works and Purposes. 1864.

White, William A. **The Principles of Mental Hygiene.** 1917.